Key advances i
the clinical manage...

of

Ovarian Cancer

Edited by

Sadaf Ghaem-Maghami, Katharine Orton
and Pat Soutter

*Proceedings of a symposium sponsored by Bristol-Myers Squibb and Schering-Plough and
held at the Royal Society of Medicine, London, 23rd January 2003*

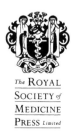

The ROYAL
SOCIETY of
MEDICINE
PRESS Limited

Published by the Royal Society of Medicine Press Ltd
1 Wimpole Street, London W1G 0AE, UK.
Tel: +44 (0)20 7290 2921; Fax: +44 (0)20 7290 2929.
Email: publishing@rsm.ac.uk
Website: www.rsmpress.co.uk

Customers in North America should order via:
RSM Press, c/o Jamco Distribution Inc., 1401 Lakeway Drive, Lewisville, TX 75057, USA.
Tel: +1 800 538 1287 (toll free); Fax: +1 972 353 1303.
Email: jamco@majors.com

These proceedings are published by the Royal Society of Medicine Press Ltd with financial support from the sponsor. The contributors are responsible for the scientific content and the views expressed, which are not necessarily those of the editors of the series or of the volume, of the Royal Society of Medicine or of the Royal Society of Medicine Press Ltd. Distribution has been in accordance with the wishes of the sponsor but a copy is available to any fellow of the society at a privileged price.

Although every effort has been made to ensure that, where provided, information concerning drug dosages or product usage has been presented accurately in this publication, the ultimate responsibility rests with the prescribing physician and neither the publisher nor the sponsor can be held responsible for errors or any consequences arising from the use of information contained herein.

British Library Cataloguing in Publication Data

A catalogue record for this book is available from the British Library

ISBN 1-85315-559-4

Typeset by Phoenix Photosetting, Chatham, Kent

Printed in Great Britain by Latimer Trend & Company Ltd, Plymouth

Editors

Dr Sadaf Ghaem-Maghami
Queen Charlotte's and Chelsea Hospital, Du Cane Road, London

Dr Katharine Orton
Council Member, Section of General Practice, RSM, London;
Hatfield Heath and Hatfield Broad Oak Surgeries, Bishop's Stortford, Hertfordshire

Mr Pat Soutter
Reader in Gynaecological Oncology,
Imperial College, Hammersmith Hospital, London

Contributors

Dr Nandita deSouza
Department of Imaging, Hammersmith Hospital, Du Cane Road, London

Professor Ian Jacobs
St Bartholomew's and The London; Queen Mary's School of Medicine, London

Professor Stanley Kaye
Royal Marsden Hospital, London

Dr Paul Pharoah
Cancer Research UK, Senior Research Fellow,
Department of Oncology, University of Cambridge

Professor Gordon Rustin
Director of Medical Oncology, Mount Vernon Hospital, Northwood, Middlesex

Dr Adrian Tookman
Royal Free Hospital NHS Trust, Edenhall Marie Curie Centre, London

Professor Michael Wells
University of Sheffield Medical School, Sheffield

Contents

Preface

Of all the female cancers, cancer of the ovary causes the most fear and loathing. This is true not only in patients and carers, but also in medical staff due to the insidious and rapid onset of the disease – women are likely to present in stage III or IV with spread beyond the ovary or the pelvis. In this book we hope to bring the reader an up-to-date picture of the medical understanding of this dreaded disease.

Over 5000 cases of ovarian cancer are diagnosed every year in the UK. Most occur in women with no known genetic mutation. Screening is being investigated as a means of detecting cases at an earlier stage. The chapter on screening describes the challenges that this poses.

Subsequent chapters follow the patient through imaging, surgery and histopathology. These allow a formal detailed tissue diagnosis to be made and further therapy can then be planned on an individual basis. The chapter on first-line chemotherapy explains the efforts being made to maximize survival while using least toxicity, particularly in early ovarian cancer. Where necessary, it is possible to offer relapse chemotherapy and symptom control to maintain an acceptable quality of life. The latest thoughts on this can be found in the final chapters.

We recommend this book to GPs, primary healthcare teams, medical students and those training in gynaecology, gynaecological oncology and palliative care as an up-to-date overview of cancer of the ovary and common controversies in its management.

S Ghaem-Maghami
K Orton
P Soutter

The role of the primary-care physician

Katharine Orton, Section of General Practice, RSM, London; Hatfield Heath and Broad Oak Surgeries, Bishop's Stortford, Hertfordshire

The role of primary care extends from the cradle to the grave, from the moment a person becomes worried about a symptom to the point of death. In the context of ovarian cancer, primary-care physicians have some responsibility for the areas of genetic risk awareness, diagnosis, referral and case management. After diagnosis, primary-care roles include maintaining the momentum of treatment, providing support during treatment, maintaining follow-up, diagnosing recurrence promptly and giving palliative care.

Most general practitioners (GPs) will see no more than one case of ovarian cancer every six years. When GPs do see ovarian cancer, they often direct their patients to the wrong place; in one centre 42.5% of 46 cases of ovarian cancer were originally referred to non-gynaecological specialties.

An ongoing study by Joan Austoker and colleagues[1] aims to find the significant diagnostic factors for ovarian cancer in primary care. The study involves interviewing three groups of women:

- New patients with ovarian cancer who appear in gynaecology clinics.
- New patients in non-gynaecology clinics who are diagnosed with ovarian cancer.
- Patients without ovarian cancer referred to a fast-track gynaecology service.

The referring GPs are also interviewed. The idea is to identify the factors that should have precipitated the diagnosis of ovarian cancer, to understand how the women expressed these symptoms and to see how these symptoms have been interpreted and then acted on by the patients and their doctors. The results of this study should help to reduce delays in presentation, referral and diagnosis. The addition of a national screening programme for ovarian cancer would, of course, also aid in the situation.

GP workload concerning ovarian cancer comes principally from worried females with a single relative who has, or had, ovarian cancer. Managing these cases sensitively, whilst knowing that they are more at risk than the rest of the population, is difficult and may necessitate referral to a gynaecologist. The families with BRCA1 and BRCA2 mutations are much rarer and need to be offered specialist follow-up – further information is given in the paper by Dr Pharoah, but the undisputed benefits of prophylactic oophorectomy in this patient group reinforces our duty to identify the families concerned.

Case study

A married woman aged 49 and with four children came to see me on the morning of Thursday 15 October 1992 because her abdomen was very distended. According to the patient there had been no distension the previous evening. She was wearing her work uniform, but the dress was so tight that she could not move it. She planned to go to work after her appointment.

The patient had experienced heartburn for about a month. She described the pain as 'being on fire' retrosternally and said it was there most of the time. She had no nausea and her bowels were open normally. Apart from a feeling of discomfort on the morning she came to see me, she claimed to feel well. On further questioning, the patient admitted that she had felt full very early on when eating during the period that she had been experiencing heartburn. She told me she was drinking large amounts of coffee, and wondered whether that was to blame for her symptoms. She volunteered the information that her mother had had carcinoma of the uterus.

On examination, the patient had difficulty in lifting her dress, having to wriggle to push it up. I sensed that she would not normally have dressed in clothing that was too tight. The patient had a bloated abdomen, and she was tender on the left side. On vaginal examination, there was a craggy mass in the left iliac fossa or left adnexae. The uterus was of normal size. The rectum contained some faeces but nothing else of note.

I arranged an ultrasound scan for the following Monday morning, 19 October. I then spoke to a consultant gynaecologist, who agreed to see the patient on 22 October. It was on the repeated ultrasound scan that our fears were confirmed – the patient had a primary ovarian carcinoma. The patient was admitted for laparotomy on 27 October and had her operation on 28 October, 13 days after presenting at my surgery. She underwent total abdominal hysterectomy and bilateral salpingo-oophorectomy and omentectomy.

On laparotomy, the surgeon found considerable ascites. There was a large, left-sided ovarian cyst, which was partly solid and partly cystic. The peritoneum of the pelvis appeared very red and inflamed. The right ovary and uterus were normal. The preoperative CA125 level was 11 600 U/ml. The ascitic fluid was positive for malignancy. Histological tests showed invasive carcinoma of the ovary of endometrioid and clear-cell variety. The omentum showed secondary deposits. The disease was classified as stage III and the patient was referred for chemotherapy.

On 6 November, the gynaecologist wrote to the oncologist to request chemotherapy. The patient was seen by the oncologist on 17 November. He said that although he did not want to delay treatment, there was a wait on the NHS. Instead, the patient was referred privately, and she had her first chemotherapy on 24 November. The patient had her first CT scan (carried out privately) on 16 December. This showed complete excision and no abnormalities of the para-aortic area. The patient returned to work in February the following year.

Ten years on, although she is now well, the patient continues by choice to see the oncologist (privately) every six months. The oncologist does a CA125 blood test and examines the patient thoroughly but does not arrange an ultrasound scan.

Conclusion

This patient did not know that there was anything wrong with her until just before she came to my surgery, which raises the question: is there any way that we can get women to sense there is something wrong earlier? Several articles have been written about how women feel when they have ovarian cancer symptoms.[2] The symptoms are often dismissed by women as being related to normal body changes, such as childbirth, menopause or stress. If we add in irritable bowel syndrome and the usual discomfort and symptoms associated with periods and the menopause, it comes as no surprise that many women with ovarian cancer do not know that something more serious is happening to them. It is often only when their symptoms become severe and include pain, as in this case, that an appointment is made to see the GP.

The primary-care team has many roles in many diseases, but somehow we have to foster an alert response to patients' symptoms. GPs often leave the first point of contact with patients to their nursing staff. Do the nursing staff know what to pick up on? Do they know any better than GPs? Are they actually even better than GPs? We cannot answer these questions generically, but we can say with certainty that the way primary care is spreading the load will make a difference to the way patients present with ovarian cancer and other diseases.

References

1. Bankhead C, Kehoe S, Austoker J on behalf of the Ovarian Symptoms and Diagnosis Study Group. Identifying potentially significant diagnostic factors for ovarian cancer in primary care: a qualitative and quantitative study. Poster presented at the national meeting of the Society for Academic Primary Care (SAPC), Birmingham, UK, July 2002.
2. Fitch M, Deane K, Howell D, Gray RE. Women's experiences with ovarian cancer: reflections on being diagnosed. Can Oncol Nurs J 2002; 12: 152–68.

The value of screening

Ian Jacobs, St Bartholomew's and The London; Queen Mary's School of Medicine, London

Patients with ovarian cancer overwhelmingly present with disease outside the ovary, ie stage II, III or IV; most present with stage III disease disseminated around the peritoneal cavity (as seen in the case study in Dr Orton's paper). Patients with disease outside the ovary have very poor five-year survival rates, but the few patients (10–15% in properly staged series) presenting with stage I disease have five-year survival rates in excess of 90% (Figure 1). If we could shift patients from the later stages of ovarian cancer to stage I,

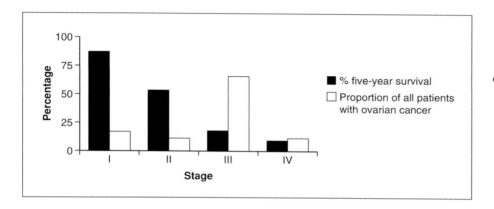

Figure 1: Current five-year survival and stage distribution for ovarian cancer.

then without altering the five-year survival rate for each stage, we may be able to increase the overall five-year survival from 30–40% to 70–80% (Figure 2).

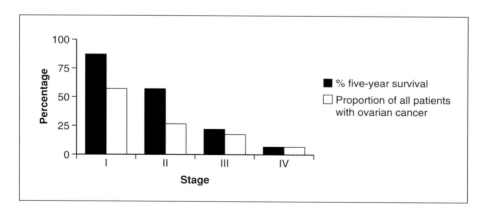

Figure 2: Potential stage shift achievable by early detection.

As only a small proportion of the population is in the high-risk familial ovarian cancer group, we are only going to have a major impact on mortality from ovarian cancer if we consider screening the general population.

Challenges of screening

Screening aims to decrease mortality by detecting preclinical disease and allowing us to intervene in early-stage ovarian cancer. However, some believe that the time interval from normal ovarian function through premalignant change and preclinical disease to invasive ovarian cancer is too short for screening to be feasible. Furthermore even if we can detect preclinical disease, this still may not save lives because all we may do is demonstrate lead-time bias or length-time bias. It may be that to effectively screen for ovarian cancer we need to identify premalignant change – analogous to cervical dysplasia – but this is not possible at the moment.

Screening is expensive; it will result in some morbidity because of false-positive operations being carried out, and it may not be acceptable to the entire population. It is important to achieve a balance between the predicted decrease in mortality and these negative aspects. Therefore, before we can carry out a randomized, controlled trial of screening, we needed to find a test that achieves:

- Very high sensitivity – at least 85–90%.
- An acceptably low number of false-positive operations for each case of ovarian cancer detected – preferably fewer than ten.

To put this into context, ovarian cancer is a relatively uncommon disease: if all postmenopausal women over age 50 in the UK are screened for ovarian cancer, then one in 2500 each year will develop ovarian cancer. To achieve fewer than 10 false-positives for each ovarian cancer detected, the test must have a minimum specificity of 99.6% (ie 0.4 of 2500 = 10).

Screening strategies

Two strategies have been investigated in many thousands of women over the past 15 years. The multimodal approach involves an initial CA125 blood test and women with abnormal tests are then asked to undergo ultrasound scanning. We pioneered this approach, starting in 1985, at St Bartholomew's Hospital and the Royal London Hospital.[1-5] A lot of work has also been done in Stockholm by Nina Einhorn's group.[6] So far, about 100 000 screens have been carried out in 50 000 women, and 28 ovarian cancers have been detected.

The other approach is to use ultrasound scanning as a first-line test. If the ultrasound is abnormal, scanning is repeated, perhaps using colour-flow. This approach has been studied by a number of groups.[7-11] These studies have involved 110 000 women, with 200 000 screens being undertaken and 47 ovarian cancers being detected.

Ultrasound screening

The first important study with ultrasound, reported in 1989, was that of Campbell and colleagues at King's College London.[7] A total of 5500 women were screened every year for three years using transabdominal ultrasound. Five ovarian cancers were detected and there were no false-negatives, ie 100% sensitivity. However, three of the cancers were borderline ovarian tumours, and intervening by screening will not change the natural history of these good prognostic tumours. The problem was that they had to operate on 326 women with abnormal ultrasound to detect the five cancers, ie there were 50 unnecessary operations for each patient detected with ovarian cancer.

Ultrasound has since been refined, with more sophisticated machines, better resolution and serial monitoring being carried out to see whether abnormalities persist. There is also recognition that simple unilocular anechoic ovarian cysts carry a very low risk for malignancy.[9] In addition, morphological indices have been developed that study the ovary and pick out high-risk morphology to determine whether surgical intervention should be performed. Combining these refinements reduces the number of false-positive operations per case of ovarian cancer to 10–15 in the best centres.[9]

Screening using tumour markers

The advantages of using tumour markers as a first-line test are that sampling can be done anywhere, it is quick and simple, the assays can all be done in one central laboratory, giving objective, reproducible results, and it is cheaper than ultrasound. This is the approach that we started working on in 1985 at the Royal London Hospital and then at St Bartholomew's Hospital.

The first phase involved a prevalence screen of 22 000 postmenopausal women over age 50. Women with a CA125 level above 30 U/ml were asked back for a transabdominal scan. An ovarian volume greater than 8.8 ml led to a referral for further assessment to determine whether or not surgery should be undertaken. This study showed that there was a very good correlation between the risk of ovarian cancer and CA125 level: a CA125 level above 30 U/ml gave a 100-fold increase in risk and if the level was above 100 U/ml, the increase in risk was 300-fold.[3]

The second issue investigated in this study was whether it is possible to intervene early enough in the natural history of ovarian cancer. A change-point model looking at the pattern of CA125 over time estimated the lead time for CA125 to be 1.9 years, and the prevalence-screen data gave a lead time of 1.5 years.[4] This provides some reassurance for the concern that the pattern of CA125 in preclinical ovarian cancer rises so steeply that we would not be able to intervene.

Of 22 000 women screened in the prevalence study, 717 had a CA125 level above 30 U/ml. Of these, 73 had an abnormal scan and went on to surgery where it was found that 19 had ovarian cancer, ie there were three false-positive operations for each ovarian cancer detected.[3] These results were good enough to proceed to the next phase of the study, which randomized the 22 000 women into either a control group (no further screening) or a study group (annual screening for three years). The women were followed for a mean of eight years, both by postal questionnaire and through the UK cancer registry. There were no differences between the groups for age, age at menarche, age at menopause, race, parity, smoking, use of the oral contraceptive pill, family history, histological type of ovarian cancer or prevalence screen results. The encouraging results of this phase were that there was a difference in median survival and in the survival curves between the study group and the control group.[4] The study was not large enough to establish whether there was a significant mortality difference, although the number of deaths from ovarian cancer in the screened group was half that in the control group.

We then tried to refine the approach to screening because the sensitivity was quite low (70%). The approach we took was to look more carefully at the CA125 patterns. Instead of using a cut-off value, we studied CA125 levels over time. In women who had a CA125 level above 30 U/ml but who did not develop ovarian cancer, the CA125 pattern is either flat or falls with time; in women who did develop ovarian cancer, the CA125 pattern almost always rises exponentially with time.[5]

We developed an algorithm to compare a woman's CA125 profile with the patterns in known cases of ovarian cancer and in healthy women. The closer the profile is to the known cases of ovarian cancer in our database, the greater the risk of developing ovarian cancer. This gives a woman's percentage risk each year of developing ovarian cancer based on her CA125 pattern. We then triaged the women into three groups:

- normal ($\leq$1/2000) risk: annual CA125 testing carried out
- elevated (>1/500) risk: woman asked back for ultrasound scan
- Intermediate (>1/2000–$\leq$1/500) risk: woman asked back for repeat CA125 testing until the pattern falls into the normal or elevated group (after three or four repeats over several months, the pattern always goes into one of these groups).

The sensitivity of this approach using our retrospective database of 50 000 samples approached 85%, analogous to ultrasound, maintaining the high specificity and the low false-positive rates.[6] As these were retrospective data, we went on to test the algorithm prospectively. This pilot trial, which finished in 2001, randomized 14 000 women to two groups. Preliminary results reveal only two false-positives for each case of ovarian cancer detected, and apparently a sensitivity of 85%.

Acceptability and economic feasibility

One of the important things we have learnt from our trials is that screening for ovarian cancer is acceptable to women. Women who had taken part in the CA125 study, and who had also undergone cervical screening, mammography and ultrasound scanning, were asked to rank the various screening tests in order of acceptability. The blood test for CA125 was considered to be the most acceptable screening test, while the acceptability of ultrasound was similar to that of cervical screening and mammography (unpublished data).

Another issue we considered in our trials was economic feasibility. The best estimate from the randomized trial of the cost per year of life saved was £12 900, which is within the bounds of acceptable healthcare interventions in the UK.

On the basis of the feasibility, acceptability, high specificity, satisfactory positive predictive value, encouraging sensitivity, preliminary evidence of a survival benefit and the possibility that we were able to reduce mortality, we received funding to undertake a very large, randomized, controlled trial – the UK Collaborative Trial of Ovarian Cancer Screening (UKCTOCS). This ongoing trial aims to randomize 200 000 postmenopausal women over age 50 into three groups:

- a multimodal group using CA125 as a primary test and ultrasound as a secondary test
- a group in which ultrasound is the primary test
- a control group.

The primary endpoint of UKCTOCS is ovarian cancer mortality. Secondary endpoints include morbidity associated with screening, health economics, quality of life, acceptability and compliance. To date over 80 000 women have been recruited and the study will report in 2010.

The future

Finally, Petricoin and colleagues, using proteomic technology, looked at the pattern of protein peaks in the serum of women with and without ovarian cancer.[12] They found five different peaks that distinguished the two groups of women. There are various problems with these preliminary data, but several similar studies that are not yet published do suggest that the power and the potential of this technology are worth investigating further.

By the time our study of screening is completed, more powerful technology will probably be available. Therefore, if we can prove that ovarian cancer screening does reduce mortality, we should soon be able to use tests with greater sensitivity.

Conclusion

Screening may fulfil the desperate need for progress in ovarian cancer, and there is a persuasive rationale for screening. There are well-defined strategies, with high specificity, high positive predictive value and encouraging sensitivity. There is evidence of lead time, so detecting early ovarian cancer may allow us to intervene and thus increase survival. Intervening with screening is feasible, economically viable and acceptable to the target population of women. We need to await the results of UKCTOCS to determine the impact of screening on mortality from ovarian cancer.

Acknowledgements

I would like to acknowledge the enormous amount of funding from a range of charities and grant-awarding bodies in the UK, including ROC, GCRF, MRC, CRUK and NHS R&D. These studies cost vast amounts of money, and a huge effort is involved. Many thousands of women and thousands of healthcare professionals have taken part in these studies, from community general practitioners and nurses through to specialist centres; I am grateful to them all, particularly my colleagues and collaborators in the trial centre at St Bartholomew's Hospital and the 13 UK centres that are taking part in UKCTOCS.

References

1. Jacobs I, Stabile I, Bridges J et al. Multimodal approach to screening for ovarian cancer. Lancet 1988; **1**: 268–71.

2. Jacobs IJ, Skates SJ, MacDonald N et al. Screening for ovarian cancer: a pilot randomised controlled trial. Lancet 1999; **353**: 1207–10.

3. Jacobs I, Davies AP, Bridges J et al. Prevalence screening for ovarian cancer in postmenopausal women by CA 125 measurement and ultrasonography. BMJ 1993; **306**: 1030–4.

4. Menon U, Talaat A, Rosenthal AN et al. Performance of ultrasound as a second line test to serum CA 125 in ovarian cancer screening. BJOG 2000; **107**: 165–9.

5. Skates SJ, Menon U, MacDonald N et al. Calculation of the Risk of Ovarian Cancer From Serial CA-125 Values for Preclinical Detection in Postmenopausal Women. J Clin Oncol 2003; **21 (10 Suppl)**: 206–10.

6. Einhorn N, Sjovall K, Knapp RC et al. Prospective evaluation of serum CA 125 levels for early detection of ovarian cancer. Obstet Gynecol 1992; **80**: 14–18.

7. Bourne TH, Campbell S, Reynolds K et al. The potential role of serum CA 125 in an ultrasound-based screening program for familial ovarian cancer. Gynecol Oncol 1994; **52**: 379–58.

8. Campbell S, Bhan V, Royston P et al. Transabdominal ultrasound screening for early ovarian cancer. BMJ 1989; **299**: 1363–7.

9. DePriest PD, van Nagell JR Jr, Gallion HH et al. Ovarian cancer screening in asymptomatic postmenopausal women. Gynecol Oncol 1993; **51**: 205–9.

10. Kurjak A, Shalan H, Kupesic S et al. An attempt to screen asymptomatic women for ovarian and endometrial cancer with transvaginal color and pulsed Doppler sonography. J Ultrasound Med 1994; **13**: 295–301.

11. Sato S, Yokoyama Y, Sakamoto T et al. Usefulness of mass screening for ovarian carcinoma using transvaginal ultrasonography. Cancer 2000; **89**: 582–8.

12. Petricoin EF, Ardekani AM, Hitt BA et al. Use of proteomic patterns in serum to identify ovarian cancer. Lancet 2002; **359**: 572–7.

Practical applications of genetics and epidemiology

Paul Pharoah, Cancer Research UK, Senior Research Fellow, Department of Oncology, University of Cambridge

Mendelian transmission of ovarian cancer was first described in the 1950s. In subsequent decades, hereditary cancer syndromes that included ovarian cancer as part of the phenotype were described. During the 1970s and 1980s, a series of observational studies reported the familial risks associated with a family history of ovarian cancer. Then in the 1990s, the genetic basis for at least part of the familial aggregation of ovarian cancer was identified.

Relevance of family history

Figure 1 puts into context the family history of ovarian cancer. The large circle represents all women with ovarian cancer. A substantial proportion of these women, as indicated by the shaded circle, also report a family history. A small fraction of those women with a family history will have an identifiable germ-line or inherited genetic abnormality. However, there is also a very small fraction of women with an identifiable abnormality who have no family history.

The observational studies carried out in the 1970s and 1980s showed that having one first-degree relative with ovarian cancer confers an approximately three-fold increase in risk. A meta-analysis by Stratton and colleagues confirmed this.[1] In the UK, a three-fold increased risk equates to about a 4% risk of ovarian cancer by age 70.

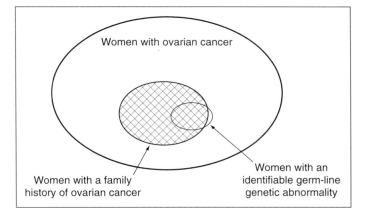

A recent study looking at the co-segregation of ovarian cancer in twins has been published. This suggested that the majority of familial aggregation is due to inherited factors rather than shared environmental factors.[2]

Figure 1: Relevance of family history.

High-penetrance ovarian cancer genes

The hereditary breast ovarian cancer syndrome was first described in the 1970s.[3] Several linkage studies that started in the 1980s localized a breast–ovarian cancer susceptibility gene to the long arm of chromosome 17, and *BRCA1* was finally isolated in 1994.[4] A second breast cancer gene, *BRCA2*, was cloned in 1995.[5] *BRCA2* was also subsequently shown to be associated with an increased risk of ovarian cancer. Ovarian cancer is also part of the characteristic phenotype of hereditary non-polyposis colorectal cancer, a syndrome caused by mutations in the family of mismatch-repair genes.

What then is the role of *BRCA1* and *BRCA2* in familial ovarian cancer? The data shown in Figure 2 come from the UK Familial Ovarian Cancer Register. Families with at least two women that are first- or second-degree relatives and are affected with ovarian cancer are eligible for the register. Women affected with breast or ovarian cancer from the 112 families on the register have been screened for mutations in the two genes.[6] The proportion of mutation-positive families is highly dependent on the strength of the familial aggregation. Almost 50 families fulfilled the criteria of (a) having four or more cases of breast and ovarian cancer or (b) having at least three ovarian cancers. Over half of these families were accounted for by *BRCA1* or *BRCA2*, the vast majority being due to *BRCA1* mutations. In a small number of families, no genetic cause could be identified.

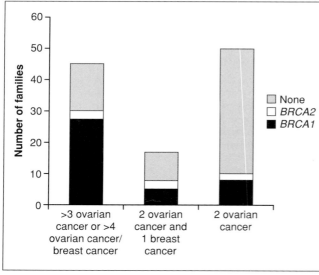

None
BRCA2
BRCA1

Figure 2: BRCA1 and BRCA2 mutation prevalence in multicase families. Adapted from Gayther et al. Am J Hum Genet 1999; 65: 1021–9.

In the slightly less strong aggregations – families with two cases of ovarian cancer and one case of breast cancer (ie three affected women/family) – less than half of the families were found to have a mutation in either *BRCA1* or *BRCA2*. Most of the families consist of just two case aggregations, ie two affected women on the same side of the family; only a small proportion of these families had *BRCA1* and *BRCA2* mutations, with the genetic cause in the remaining families being unknown.

The prevalence of *BRCA1* mutations in ovarian cancer cases unselected for family history has been reported by four studies.[7-11] The first published study found 12 truncating mutations in 374 cases (3%) from Southern England.[8] A subsequent larger study reported a higher prevalence, with 39 mutations in 515 patients (8%) from Canada.[11] However, a substantial proportion of these mutations were in cases from the Ashkenazi Jewish or French Canadian ethnic groups, in whom common founder mutations are known to be prevalent. In the 316 cases of British origin, only 8 (2.5%) were *BRCA1* mutation carriers. The other two studies, both from the USA, were smaller: one reported 10 mutations in 116 patients[9] and the other found four mutations in 120 cases.[12]

Less data are available for *BRCA2*, but the Canadian study reported 21 truncating mutations out of a total of 515 cases (4%) of which seven occurred in the 316 cases of British origin (2.2% prevalence). The study reported by Rubin *et al* found only one *BRCA2* mutation carrier in 116 cases.[9]

Risks associated with *BRCA1* and *BRCA2* mutations

Figures 3 and 4 show the age-associated cumulative risk of cancer associated with *BRCA1* and *BRCA2* mutations. The estimate of risk depends on how it is determined. For *BRCA1*, the breast cancer risk estimated using data derived from multicase families is 85% by age 70, but in studies that used pedigree from mutation carriers identified in case series unselected for family history, the breast cancer risk is somewhat lower. The risk of ovarian cancer estimated from multicase families is also high (60% by age 70), but again the risk estimate is lower when data from case series unselected for family history are used.

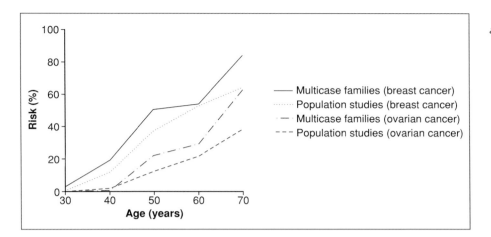

Figure 3: Risk associated with BRCA1 mutation.

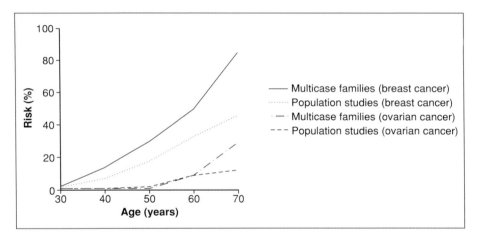

Figure 4: Risk associated with BRCA2 mutation.

For *BRCA2*, the risk of breast cancer is very high when multicase families are used to estimate penetrance, but the risk is somewhat lower when unselected case series are used. For ovarian cancer, *BRCA2* clearly has a lower penetrance than *BRCA1*. When the population-based study is used, the ovarian cancer penetrance is as low as 10–15% by age 70.

The differences in the mutation-associated penetrance estimates suggest that there are modifiers of risk that segregate within families; these may be either genetic or lifestyle/environmental. Several studies are currently looking for genetic modifiers of risk; although various possibilities have been reported, there is as yet no definitive evidence for a genetic modifier. Increasing evidence is available to explain some environmental modifiers of risk,[13] although the data are still somewhat sparse.

Oral contraceptive pill

There has been a large amount of interest in how use of the oral contraceptive pill (OCP) might modify both breast and ovarian cancer risk in mutation carriers. One of the first studies from the USA showed that using the pill reduced the risk of developing ovarian cancer by more than 50%.[14] This reduction in risk is similar to that in the general population, but a subsequent study from Israel showed no reduction in risk of ovarian cancer with use of the pill.[15] However, differences in the year of birth between cases and controls and variations in pill usage over time might have accounted for the negative findings in the Israeli study.

We have combined data from the UK register with data from a similar register in the USA. Although the results of this study have not been published yet, we found a 40% reduction in risk of developing ovarian cancer associated with a past history of oral contraceptive use.

For breast cancer, the effect of the pill in mutation carriers is unclear, but there are suggestions that its use increases the risk of breast cancer. Large studies are currently under way to clear up the controversies surrounding the effect of OCP use on breast and ovarian cancer risk.

Prophylactic oophorectomy

The one thing that is incontrovertible in terms of risk reduction for *BRCA1/BRCA2* mutation carriers is prophylactic oophorectomy, although residual ovarian epithelium in the peritoneum does leave some risk. Two papers published in 2002 showed that oophorectomy confers a substantial risk reduction. In the first study, 98 women who had undergone bilateral salpingo-oophorectomy were compared with women who had undergone ovarian cancer surveillance. The authors estimated that the risk of ovarian cancer after prophylactic oophorectomy was reduced by 85%, although the confidence intervals on their hazard ratios were rather wide due to the relatively small size of the study. They also showed, encouragingly, that oophorectomy reduces the risk of breast cancer in mutation carriers.

The second, larger study compared surveillance with oophorectomy.[16] The authors found an even bigger reduction in the risk of ovarian cancer with oophorectomy, which was highly significant. They also found a significant reduction in the risk of breast cancer.

Timing of prophylactic surgery

The risks and benefits of prophylactic surgery must be considered on an individual basis. For mutation carriers, the risk of ovarian cancer before age 40 is small, so the benefits of ovarian surgery before then are also likely to be modest. From then on, there is a fairly substantial annual risk increase of about 1.5% per year.

The negative consequences of oophorectomy related to premature menopause tend to be exaggerated, but issues regarding fertility must be considered. Thus, the most appropriate age for a woman to undergo prophylactic oophorectomy is a personal choice and depends on the relative weight that each woman places on the benefits and risks.

Clinical features of *BRCA1*-associated ovarian cancer

Ovarian cancer associated with the *BRCA1* gene has some characteristic features. In particular, it tends to be high-grade serous (non-mucinous) adenocarcinoma. Molecular studies have shown that the gene expression pattern of *BRCA1*-associated ovarian cancer has a particular signature. However, the clinical relevance of this is not clear. For example, the results of several studies comparing *BRCA1* mutation carriers with ovarian cancer patients in general have not shown convincingly that prognosis is dependent on mutation status. As yet, there is no rationale for treating women with mutations differently from any other ovarian cancer case.

Risks in ovarian cancer families with no identifiable *BRCA1* or *BRCA2* mutation

The cancer risks for women in multi-case ovarian cancer families where no *BRCA1* or *BRCA2* mutation has been identified are estimated less well than for women with a known mutation. Furthermore, the effects of modifiers are unknown, and the benefits of intervention are poorly understood. Figure 5 shows the cumulative risk of ovarian cancer according to type of family history. This shows that the risks may be substantial depending on the degree of family history. In multi-case, mutation-negative families the breast cancer risks are also fairly high, so the women are at substantial risk of disease even when no mutation has been identified.

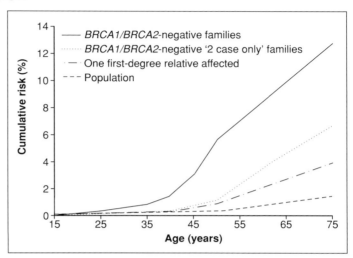

Figure 5: Cumulative risk of ovarian cancer by family history – BRCA1 or BRCA2 mutation-negative families with only two cases of ovarian cancer.

Management of women with family history of ovarian cancer

As with most other familial cancers, management is dependent on risk stratification; in this case into women at high and low risk of ovarian cancer. The group of women at high risk should be divided into those for whom it would be appropriate to refer for specialist management by a clinical geneticist, and those who should be managed within a secondary-care setting. Women who are deemed to be at relatively low risk are usually reassured to find that their risk is not substantial.

When determining whether a patient is at high or low risk based on family history, it is important to include only women with invasive ovarian cancer. High-risk women are those with:

- one first-degree relative with *invasive* ovarian cancer diagnosed at any age and one first-degree relative with breast cancer diagnosed before the age of 50 years
- two first- or second-degree relatives with *confirmed invasive* ovarian cancer at any age.

In high-risk families it may be appropriate to discuss the options and the pros and cons of oophorectomy with the first-degree female relatives of affected women. Where possible, women at high risk should be entered into a screening study.

The criteria for genetic testing vary across the UK, so there are no hard and fast rules. However, the following criteria are often used to identify families in whom a search for a mutation in *BRCA1* and/or *BRCA2* may be carried out:

- four or more relatives diagnosed at any age with invasive ovarian or breast cancer
- two or more first-degree relatives diagnosed with invasive ovarian cancer
- one first-degree relative diagnosed at any age with ovarian cancer, and two first-degree relatives diagnosed with breast cancer before age 60
- one relative diagnosed at any age with both breast and ovarian cancer.

The management of women undergoing genetic testing is done within the specialist setting of a cancer genetics clinic.

Conclusion

BRCA1 and *BRCA2* account for about one-half of familial ovarian cancers with at least two cases in the family. The risk of ovarian cancer is much higher in *BRCA1* mutation carriers than in *BRCA2* mutation carriers. Some understanding of the risk modifiers is beginning to emerge, but it is important to remember that there are substantial ovarian and breast cancer risks in women from mutation-negative families. Clearly, we need more precise estimates of risk in defined subgroups, but there are no absolutes when it comes to interpreting risk.

References

1. Stratton JF, Pharoah PDP, Smith SK *et al.* A systematic review and meta-analysis of family history and risk of ovarian cancer. *Br J Obstet Gynaecol* 1998; **105**: 493–9.

2. Lichtenstein P, Holm NV, Verkasalo PK *et al.* Environmental and heritable factors in the causation of cancer – analyses of cohorts of twins from Sweden, Denmark and Finland. *N Engl J Med* 2000; **343**: 78–85.

3. Lynch HT, Guirgis HA, Albert S *et al.* Familial association of carcinoma of the breast and ovary. *Surg Gynecol Obstet* 1974; **138**: 717–24.

4. Miki Y, Swensen J, Shattuck-Eidens D *et al.* A strong candidate for the 17 linked breast and ovarian cancer susceptibility gene BRCA1. *Science* 1994; **266**: 66–71.

5. Wooster R, Bignell G, Lancaster J *et al.* Identification of the breast cancer susceptibility gene BRCA2. *Nature* 1995; **378**: 789–92.

6. Gayther SA, de Foy KA, Harrington P *et al.* The frequency of germline mutations in the breast cancer predisposition genes BRCA1 and BRCA2 in familial prostate cancer. The Cancer Research Campaign/British Prostate Group United Kingdom Familial Prostate Cancer Study Collaborators. *Cancer Res* 2000; **60**: 4513–18.

7. Matsushima M, Kobayashi K, Emi M *et al.* Mutation analysis of the BRCA1 gene in 76 Japanese ovarian cancer patients: four germline mutations, but no evidence of somatic mutation. *Hum Mol Genet* 1995; **4**: 1953–6.

8. Stratton JF, Gayther SA, Russell P *et al.* Contribution of BRCA1 mutations to ovarian cancer. *N Engl J Med* 1997; **336**: 1125–30.

9. Rubin SC, Blackwood MA, Bandera C *et al.* BRCA1, BRCA2 and hereditary nonpolyposis colorectal cancer gene mutations in an unselected ovarian cancer population: relationship to family history and implications for genetic testing. *Am J Obstet Gynecol* 1998; **178**: 670–7.

10. Janezic SA, Ziogas A, Krumroy LM *et al.* Germline BRCA1 alterations in a population-based series of ovarian cancer cases. *Hum Mol Genet* 1999; **8**: 889–97.

11. Risch HA, McLaughlin JR, Cole DE *et al.* Prevalence and penetrance of germline BRCA1 and BRCA2 mutations in a population series of 649 women with ovarian cancer. *Am J Hum Genet* 2001; **68**: 700–10.

12. Anton-Culver HA, Cohen PF, Gildea ME, Ziogas A. Characteristics of BRCA1 mutations in a population-based case series of breast and ovarian cancer. *Eur J Cancer* 2000; **36**: 1200–8.

13. Narod SA. Modifiers of risk of hereditary breast and ovarian cancer. *Nat Rev Cancer* 2002; **2**: 113–23.

14. Narod SA, Risch H, Moslehi R *et al.* Oral contraceptives and the risk of hereditary ovarian cancer. *N Engl J Med* 1998; **339**: 424–8.

15. Modan B, Hartge P, Hirsh-Yechezkel G *et al.* Parity, oral contraceptives and the risk of ovarian cancer among carriers and noncarriers of a BRCA1 or BRCA2 mutation. *N Engl J Med* 2001; **345**: 235–40.

16. Rebbeck TR, Lynch HT, Neuhausen SL *et al.* Prophylactic oophorectomy in carriers of BRCA1 or BRCA2 mutations. *N Engl J Med* 2002; **346**: 1616–22.

The role of imaging

Nandita deSouza, Hammersmith Hospital, London

Imaging in ovarian cancer is required to inform decision-makers in the clinical management of the disease and includes disease detection, characterization, staging, assessment of response to therapy and assessment of recurrence. A number of imaging modalities are available, including ultrasound with Doppler, computerized tomography (CT), magnetic resonance (MR) (mainly magnetic resonance imaging [MRI], as the efficacy of magnetic resonance spectroscopy [MRS] has not been proven in ovarian cancer) and positron-emission tomography (PET). Combination modalities are becoming increasingly popular, ranging from the laborious co-registration of image data sets in which functional information is overlaid on anatomical information, to the newer, combined CT-PET and MR-PET machines, the utility of which remains to be proven. In addition, the emerging techniques of molecular imaging that use PET, MR and optical imaging are finding their way into human clinical trials.

Technical issues

Technical issues must be addressed if the imaging examination is to be successful. Correct patient preparation is vital in order to achieve images of diagnostic quality. Patient preparation varies with the imaging examination being undertaken, but parameters such as the state of hydration or fasting of the patient, empty versus full bladder, the use of antiperistaltic agents and the administration of oral, rectal or intravenous contrast agents are all crucial. There are also issues regarding equipment capability and the best scanning protocols to optimize the spatial and temporal resolution of the images.

Transabdominal ultrasound, which uses a 3.5–5.0 MHz transducer, is utilized for assessment of abdominal and pelvic lymph nodes, renal obstruction and liver metastases. Endovaginal sonography using a 5.0–7.5 MHz probe is superior for lesions near the vaginal vault. Colour-flow and duplex Doppler imaging may be used with either probe: the former assesses vascularity while the latter can be used to characterize waveform patterns and resistive indices.

With CT, the scanned field ranges from the dome of the diaphragm to the inguinal region; it may also include the chest. Contrast opacification of the bowel is mandatory; 8–10 mm and 5 mm slice reconstruction through the abdomen and pelvis, respectively, is optimal. Intravenous contrast opacification aids differentiation between the vessels and lymph nodes.

With MRI, the use of multiple imaging planes is a distinct advantage; T2-weighted images provide maximal tissue contrast. To reduce bowel motion, the patient may be asked to remain nil-by-mouth for four to six hours before scanning. In addition, glucagon or hyoscine butylbromide may be administered intramuscularly before scanning. The use of a phased-array multicoil wrapped around the pelvis markedly improves signal-to-noise ratios and hence image quality. Respiratory motion may be controlled with respiratory triggering and vascular motion may be controlled with the use of presaturation bands, which saturate out the signal from the flowing blood.

In radioimmunoscintigraphy, monoclonal antibodies or antibody fragments are radiolabelled with a gamma-emitter such as ^{99m}Tc, ^{131}I, ^{123}I or [111]In. If ^{131}I or ^{123}I is employed, oral potassuim iodide is given to block thyroid uptake of free radioactive iodide. Blood pool subtraction techniques are required for ^{131}I studies (but not for ^{123}I or ^{111}In) to simulate the non-tumour distribution of labelled antibody. False-positive ^{131}I-imaging can arise from incomplete subtraction of radio-iodide in the urinary bladder. ^{111}In-labelled antibody has a different biodistribution, with uptake in the reticuloendothelial system, limiting its use for detection of liver metastases.

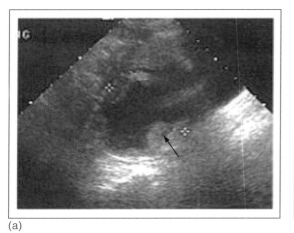

(a)

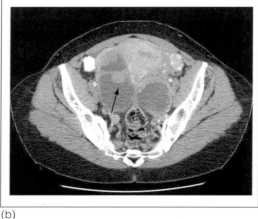

(b)

Figure 1: Bilateral complex pelvic masses: (a) ultrasound scan, showing complex cystic mass with peripheral nodular plaque (arrow); (b) CT scan, showing that the cystic masses are bilateral and contain septations and nodules (arrow).

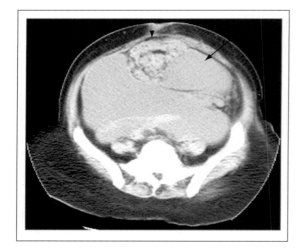

Figure 2: Metastatic spread in the abdomen: CT scan showing ascites (arrow) and omental cake (arrowhead).

Detection of disease

Imaging is essential for establishing the diagnosis of ovarian cancer by detecting a typical pelvic mass. This can be widened to encompass imaging as a screening tool. Investigations such as CT, MR and PET are not indicated for screening because of their high costs and low throughput. The only viable imaging modality for ovarian cancer screening is ultrasound. Standard greyscale imaging may be used to detect architectural changes, while vascular alterations can be detected using Doppler. Colour Doppler imaging is based on the principle that fast-growing tumours contain many new blood vessels that have relatively little smooth muscle in their walls. The resistance to flow within these vessels is therefore less than that within benign lesions. However, clinical studies have revealed that physiological changes in the premenopausal ovary at the time of ovulation have low impedance characteristics similar to those of malignancy, making the differentiation of malignant and benign lesions difficult.[1] Also, the variation in ovarian vascularity, for example pre- and post-menopause, obese patient habitus and in overlying bowel reduces the sensitivity and specificity of the technique, and its use as a screening modality in isolation remains unproven. Typically a pulsatility index of less than 1.0 and a resistive index of less than 0.4 are used to indicate malignancy.[2] The recognition of a diastolic notch can also be useful to confirm benign lesions.[2]

The constellation of a complex cystic pelvic mass with ascites, omental cake, mesenteric deposits and pleural effusions is virtually diagnostic of ovarian cancer (Figures 1 and 2). The complexity of the mass is crucial in diagnosing malignancy and may be recognized on ultrasound and CT by the presence of solid elements, septations and nodules. In the presence of a complex mass, even when there are no secondary features, malignancy is likely. A cyst with no secondary features is likely to be benign (a simple cyst or a cystadenoma). However, in addition to the complex architectural features of the lesion, lesion size alone is related directly to risk of malignancy. For primarily cystic lesions, smaller lesions carry a low risk while lesions larger than 10 cm have a 63% risk.[3]

MRI is currently underused, but it is extremely helpful in determining characteristics of the mass that are indicative of malignancy. These features are best demonstrated on T2-weighted imaging, in which loculations, septations and nodules are seen. A particular advantage of MRI over CT is that multiple planes and obliques can be used for image acquisition, including three-dimensional imaging.

PET does not contribute to determining the malignancy of pelvic masses and is not indicated for assessment of the primary mass. In a series of 99 asymptomatic pelvic masses, Fenchel and colleagues showed a significant difference in sensitivity between ultrasound and PET (Table 1).[4] This was mainly because PET gave false-positive results from benign tumours and from radioisotope within the bowel and the ureter. Low-grade T1 stage tumours also gave false-negative results with PET. Magnetic resonance imaging, although slightly less sensitive than ultrasound, was much more specific. Analysis of symptomatic complex pelvic masses in 93 patients with suspected ovarian cancer who were scheduled for surgical staging indicates that while ultrasound performs relatively well compared with MRI (sensitivity ultrasound 85%, MRI 89%), MRI had a better negative predictive value (NPV) (NPV ultrasound 73%, MRI 89%) and should be used as a problem-solving modality in complex adnexal masses.[5]

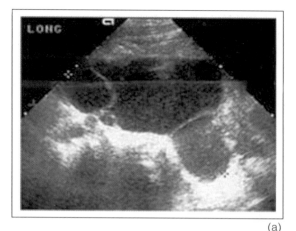

(a)

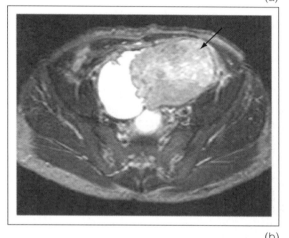

(b)

Figure 3: Ovarian cancer: (a) ultrasound scan, showing complex pelvic mass with solid and cystic components; (b) CT scan, showing that the extensive, solid component of the tumour (arrow) and more modest cystic areas. This is a clear-cell cancer, which is more solid and less mucin-producing than a cystadenocarcinoma.

Table 1 Comparison of imaging modalities in detection of ovarian cancer

	Ultrasound	MRI	PET	All three
Sensitivity (%)	92	83	58	92
Specificity (%)	60	84	76	85

Adapted from Fenchel *et al.*[4] *Radiology* 2002; **223**: 780–8.

Characterization of atypical pathology

Imaging may also be used to refine the diagnosis of complex adnexal mass in order to characterize the nature of benign or malignant lesions and identify features associated with unusual pathology. This is where MRI excels, because of the ability to manipulate image contrast with the various pulse sequences and characterize the solid compared with the cystic component of the tumour. For example, a clear-cell cancer that is less mucin-producing than a cystadenocarcinoma may be recognized by a predominantly solid mass

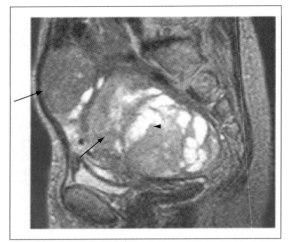

Figure 4: Granulosa cell ovarian cancer: sagittal T2-weighted MRI scan, showing a primarily solid, well-defined ovarian tumour without ascites. The mass is homogeneous, of intermediate signal intensity (arrows), with peripheral areas of cystic necrosis (arrowhead).

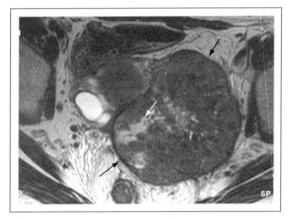

Figure 5: Malignant teratoma: transverse T2-weighted MR imaging scan shows a low signal intensity, well-defined solid mass in the left adnexa (black arrows) with central necrosis (white arrow).

with more modest cystic elements (Figure 3). Other solid tumours of the ovary include granulosa cell tumours (Figure 4) and immature teratomas (Figure 5). Different anticytokeratin monoclonal antibodies may help in distinguishing a primary ovarian adenocarcinoma from a metastatic adenocarcinoma, especially of colorectal origin.[6] Studies have also investigated the value of anti-alpha inhibin and CD99 in the diagnosis of ovarian sex cord stromal tumours.[7]

Occasionally, complex masses are benign; this is also recognized by characterizing the solid component on MRI. Well-defined, very low signal-intensity masses on T2-weighted scans are seen in cystadenofibromas (Figure 6), while mature teratomas show fat content (Figure 7). On MRI, the Short Tau Inversion Recovery (STIR) sequence nulls the signal from fat and is used to confirm the fat content of these lesions. Its use in premenopausal women is preferred over CT as it avoids radiation to the pelvis. Inflammatory masses may also present as complex adnexal cysts. In such cases, the presentation with pyrexia, pain and often a history of intrauterine device or recent intervention are key in making the diagnosis.

Disease staging

Imaging must assess the primary adnexal masses, ascites, metastases (omental cake, serosal and peritoneal deposits in pelvic and extrapelvic sites, liver deposits, lymph node enlargement) and any unresectable disease. A multi-institutional study in the USA involving several cancer sites within the body analysed prospectively 280 cases of suspected ovarian cancer and compared utility of the various imaging modalities at disease staging.[8] The conclusion was that for assessing peritoneal disease, CT and MRI were both vastly superior to ultrasound. However, the implant size in the study was greater than 2 cm rather than the subcentimeter peritoneal seedlings that are more frequently seen. Surprisingly, for lymph node and liver metastases, both CT and MRI performed poorly. An antibody to CA125 has also been widely assessed in monitoring disease extent using scintigraphy[9,10] but is limited by antibody specificity, stability and immunoreactivity, as well as patient reaction.

Assessment of response to treatment

The timing of the examination in relation to treatment is crucial. In those cases selected for interval debulking, imaging before surgery is invaluable. Imaging on completion of chemotherapy is also indicated to assess response.

Assessment of disease recurrence

Imaging can be used to assess the extent of recurrence, its resectability and its suitability for other management options. Patients with a small, isolated pelvic recurrence may be considered for pelvic exenteration. In these cases, it is often desirable to complement standard CT images with MRI or even endovaginal MRI to delineate lesion margins and attachment to neighbouring structures clearly.

MRI is also used to exclude pelvic recurrence in high-risk patients because identification and characterization of the ovarian lesion is superior with MRI. Extrapelvic recurrence is best assessed using standard CT scans that include the chest.

The role of PET in assessing disease recurrence is controversial. The key is appropriate patient selection. In patients with elevated CA 125 levels, PET can be useful because of its whole body coverage; in one small study, PET was shown to have 95% sensitivity.[11] Cho and colleagues looked at a small group of patients with epithelial ovarian cancer and suspected recurrence who had imaging before second-look laparotomy.[12] They showed that overall CT was equivalent to PET, but for nodules measuring 3–7 mm CT was superior and there was little or no advantage in using combined CT-PET.

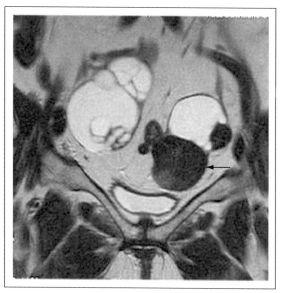

Figure 6: Benign fibrocystadenomas: coronal T2-weighted MRI scan, showing bilateral, complex, well-defined adnexal cysts with no ascites, omental cake or extrapelvic disease. The solid components (arrow) are homogeneous and very low in signal intensity, and appear fibroid in nature.

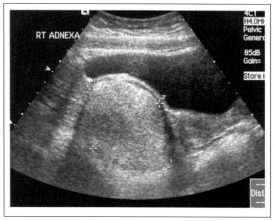

(a)

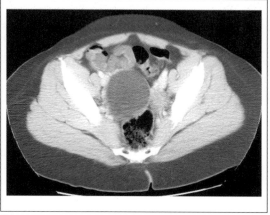

(b)

Figure 7: Dermoid: (a) ultrasound scan, showing a homogeneous, high-reflectivity, well-defined mass; (b) CT scan, showing density to be the same as that of fat, confirming that it represents a benign dermoid (mature teratoma).

Future perspectives

Emerging techniques, such as molecular imaging, aim to image specific proteins, RNA and DNA, which are orders of magnitude smaller than the overall structure and function of tissues imaged with the techniques described above. These new techniques aim to assess the efficacy of gene therapy by determining the biological action(s) of gene products and thus defining the location and magnitude of gene expression. This hinges on the detection of enzymatic reactions at a cellular level and adopts two different strategies: the use of 'smart' contrast agents and the detection of cellular accumulation of marker metabolites using PET or MRS.

Smart contrast agents have been developed for MRI that can be cleaved by enzymatic action, changing their relaxation properties so that they show significant changes in signal intensity.[13] For example, the smart contrast agent E-gad when exposed to the marker enzyme beta-galactosidase has galactopyranose removed from its cage of chelators; this transforms it from a weak to a strong relaxivity state.

A gene may be introduced and its expression imaged by monitoring the accumulation of marker metabolites. If this gene were linked to a therapeutic gene, then imaging its expression would indicate expression of the therapeutic gene. Thus, herpes simplex virus thymidine kinase (HSV-Tk) may be introduced with an adenovirus vector and its expression imaged by administering an ^{18}F-ganciclovir prodrug. The prodrug is taken up, phosphorylated by HSV-Tk and trapped intracellularly; it may then be imaged using PET.[14] In ovarian cancer models, adenovirus vectors engineered to contain HSV-Tk or somatostatin receptors have been used. The latter can be imaged using a technetium-labelled somatostatin analogue.[15] These studies are now entering pilot human clinical trials.

Magnetic resonance spectroscopy can also be used to detect gene expression by detecting changes in metabolite levels of specific marker substrates. These can take the form of prodrugs or specifically designed compounds that will be metabolized or synthesized by the marker enzyme. This approach has been utilized to detect cytosine deaminase transgene expression.[16]

Conclusion

Imaging is key in ovarian cancer for disease detection, characterization, staging, monitoring of response to treatment and assessment of recurrence. A broad spectrum of available imaging modalities must be used appropriately to answer specific questions. This calls for assessment in regional centres using available expertise and equipment.

Acknowledgements

I would like to thank our team at Hammersmith Hospital, London, in the departments of histopathology, radiology, gynaecology, oncology and palliative care, including the clerical and administrative staff involved in the care of these patients.

References

1. Carter JR, Lau M, Fowler JM *et al.* Blood flow characteristics of ovarian tumors: implications for ovarian cancer screening. *Am J Obstet Gynecol* 1995; **172**: 901–7.

2. Creasman W, DiSaia P. Screening in ovarian cancer. *Am J Obstet Gynecol* 1991; **165**: 7–10.

3. Rulin MC, Preston AL. Adnexal masses in post-menopausal women. *Obstet Gynecol* 1987; **70**: 578–81.

4. Fenchel S, Grab D, Nuessle K *et al.* Asymptomatic adnexal masses: correlation of FDG PET and histopathologic findings. *Radiology* 2002; **223**: 780–8.

5. Huber S, Medl M, Baumann L, Czembirek H. Value of ultrasound and magnetic resonance imaging in the preoperative evaluation of suspected ovarian masses. *Anticancer Res* 2002; **22**: 2501–7.

6. McCluggage WG. Recent advances in immunohistochemistry in the diagnosis of ovarian neoplasms. *J Clin Pathol* 2000;**53**: 327–34.

7. Choi YL, Kim HS, Ahn G. Immunosuppression of inhibin alpha subunit, inhibin/activin betaA subunit and CD99 in ovarian tumours. *Arch Pathol Lab Med* 2000; **124**: 563–9.

8. Tempany CMC, Zou KH, Silverman SG *et al.* Staging of advanced ovarian cancer: comparison of imaging modalities – report from the Radiological Diagnostic Oncology Group. *Radiology* 2000; **215**: 761–7.7.

9. Fayers PM, Rustin G, Wood R. The prognostic value of serum CA125 in patients with advanced ovarian carcinoma: an analysis of 573 patients by the Medical Research Council Working Party on Gynaecological Cancer. *Int J Gynaecol Cancer* 1993; **3**: 283–4

10. Surwit EA, Childers JM, Krag DN *et al.* Clinical assessment if 111 In-CYT-103 immunoscrintigraphy in ovarian cancer. *Gynecol Oncol* 1993; **48**: 285–92.

11. Chang WC, Hung YC, Kao CH *et al.* Usefulness of whole body positron emission tomography (PET) with 18F-fluoro-2-deoxyglucose (FDG) to detect recurrent ovarian cancer based on asymptomatically elevated serum levels of tumor marker. *Neoplasma* 2002; **49**: 329–33.

12. Cho SM, Ha HK, Byun JY *et al.* Usefulness of FDG PET for assessment of early recurrent epithelial ovarian cancer. *Am J Roentgenol* 2002; **179**: 391–5.

13. Szczepaniak LS, Sargeson A, Creasei II *et al.* Nuclear magnetic spin-lattice relaxation of water protons caused by metal cage compounds. *Bioconjug Chem* 1992; **3**: 27–31.

14. Gambhir SS, Barrio JR, Phelps ME *et al.* Imaging adenoviral-directed reporter gene expression in living animals with positron emission tomography. *Proc Natl Acad Sci USA* 1999: **96**: 2333–8.

15. Hemminki A, Zinn KR, Liu B *et al.* In vivo molecular chemotherapy and noninvasive imaging with an infectivity-enhanced adenovirus. *J Natl Cancer Inst* 2002; **94**: 741–9.

16. Stegman LD, Rehemtulla A, Beattie B *et al.* Non-invasive quantitation of cytosine deaminase transgene expression in human tumour xenografts with in vivo magnetic resonance spectroscopy. *Proc Natl Acad Sci USA* 1999; **96**: 9821–6.

The changing role of surgical treatment

Pat Soutter, Imperial College, Hammersmith Hospital, London

Surgery in ovarian cancer can be divided into primary cytoreductive surgery, intervention debulking, second look (which is used only rarely nowadays) and surgery for recurrent disease. Primary surgery is divided further into that for early disease, borderline tumours, germ-cell tumours and women with advanced disease.

Primary debulking surgery

The first aim of surgery in patients with ovarian cancer is to confirm the diagnosis. Although there are ways of taking biopsies, fine-needle aspirates and true-cut biopsies of masses through the abdomen, there is always a risk of disseminating the disease. Laparoscopy in a woman with advanced disease runs the risk of damaging bowel fixed by a tumour. Open laparotomy is the preferred option. In addition, an operation is often required to determine the anatomical origin of a large tumour spread diffusely throughout the peritoneum.

The second aim of surgery is to remove the entire tumour, leaving only microscopic disease. In early stage invasive disease this will be curative. In advanced disease, the hope is that this will help to relieve the patient's symptoms and that it will facilitate chemotherapy.

Borderline tumours

Borderline tumours of the ovary contain malignant epithelium that does not invade the underlying stroma of the ovary. Borderline tumours account for 10% of all epithelial tumours of the ovary. They tend to occur in young women, they are often unilateral Stage I disease, and before surgery they are often thought to be benign. Such tumours are treated entirely with surgery; there is no place for chemotherapy in the treatment of these women. Because these tumours are often thought to be benign, they are frequently treated by ovarian cystectomy. However, the recurrence rate after this is quite high (36%).[1] After cystectomy in which a borderline tumour is found unexpectedly, one has to decide between (a) re-operating to remove the rest of the ovary and (b) watching the patient carefully and waiting to see whether it recurs.

Results are better after unilateral salpingo-oophorectomy (15% recurrence) and better still with total abdominal hysterectomy and bilateral salpingo-oophorectomy (2% recurrence).[2]

Such high recurrence rates with relatively conservative therapy may sound worrying, but most of these recurrences are of borderline tumour and do not imply progression to invasive disease, which occurs only rarely. When borderline tumours recur, it is usually possible to treat them surgically with good results.[2] Ultimately, the long-term disease-free survival is excellent (Table 1).

Table 1 Survival of women with borderline tumour[2]

Stage	Disease-free survival (median 70 months' follow-up) (%)
I	99.6
II	95.8
III	89.0

Germ-cell tumours

Germ-cell tumours tend to occur in teenagers and young women, so fertility is a pressing issue. The tumours are usually unilateral and are very chemosensitive. Treatment involves careful surgical staging followed by fertility-sparing surgery. Adjuvant chemotherapy is used only in those patients with residual or recurrent disease. Secondary cytoreductive surgery might be appropriate in patients who have inadequate initial surgery or who recur after chemotherapy.

Stage I epithelial ovarian cancer

Apart from the degree of differentiation, the histopathology of epithelial cancers offers little in the way of prognostic factors. Although controversial, there is evidence from a large series that if the tumour has ruptured before surgery, then the prognosis is likely to be worse.[3] Rupture of the tumour during surgery probably worsens the prognosis.[3] The FIGO staging system is also important in determining the prognosis of early-stage ovarian disease. Women with stage I epithelial tumours may be divided in to low-risk or high-risk on the basis of the degree of differentiation, the stage and whether or not the tumour has ruptured (Table 2). This guides the advice given on the most appropriate form of treatment.

Table 2 Low- and high-risk groups for stage I epithelial ovarian cancer

	Low-risk	High-risk
Differentiation	Good or moderate	Poor
Ruptured?	No	Yes
Stage	Ia (?Ib)	Ib or Ic
Surgery	Unilateral salpingo-oophorectomy	Total abdominal hysterectomy, bilateral salpingo-oophorectomy and omentectomy
Chemotherapy?	No	Yes

Advanced epithelial ovarian cancer

Sadly, we tend to see advanced stage II and III cancers most commonly. In these women, it is important when operating to explore the abdomen carefully to confirm that this is indeed a tumour that has arisen from the ovary, to determine its extent and to perform a total abdominal hysterectomy and bilateral salpingo-oophorectomy, trying to remove any residual metastatic masses. Generally, bowel resection should be avoided (except to overcome obstruction) because this probably does not improve the prognosis. Some believe that lymphadenectomy is beneficial, but this still has to be proven.

Figure 1 depicts the results of a study by Griffiths and colleagues in 1979,[4] which showed that women with small tumours had the same prognosis as women with much larger tumours which were reduced by surgery to a small amount of residual disease. This and later studies

*Figure 1: Results of cytoreductive surgery. Adapted from Griffiths et al. Cancer Treat Rep 1979; **63**: 235–40.*

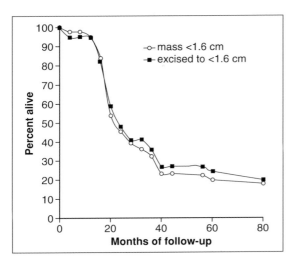

suggested that cytoreductive surgery would indeed improve the prognosis of all women with advanced ovarian disease.

However, in a meta-analysis that included a vast number of patients treated in a large number of studies of ovarian cancer surgery, it was found that while the use of platinum chemotherapy undoubtedly improved the prognosis, the effect of cytoreductive surgery did not appear to be very great.[5]

It is difficult to show an effect of surgery alone, as it is not possible to design a randomized trial that offers surgery to one group but not to the other. It seems likely that several factors are working together, including the tumour biology, the chemotherapy and the surgery. Cytoreductive surgery can give symptomatic relief and improves the tolerance of subsequent chemotherapy.

Intervention debulking

The first randomized trial to show that surgery could make a difference was a study of intervention debulking.[6] Patients who had unresected bulky disease were randomized to either intervention debulking or conventional management. The intervention debulking group were given three courses of chemotherapy. Providing their disease did not get any worse, they underwent further cytoreductive surgery (performed by the surgeon who did the first operation), followed by further chemotherapy. A total of 425 women were included in the trial. Figure 2 shows the results of the trial. The women who underwent intervention debulking surgery did marginally better than those who did not have debulking surgery and this benefit seems to continue in the longer-term follow-up.[6]

Cytoreduction versus intervention debulking

In the clinic, we are faced daily with the choice between undertaking primary cytoreductive surgery or intervention debulking. If the tumour is obviously resectable, is in the pelvis, is small in volume, is confined to stage II or III, and if there is very little upper abdominal disease, then primary cytoreduction is probably the better option. Interval debulking should be reserved for women with unresectable tumours, women with large-volume disease and women with stage IV disease where the disease has spread beyond the ovaries.

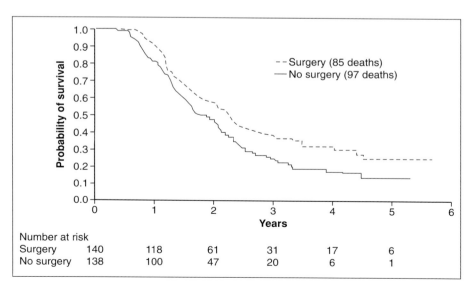

Figure 2: Results of intervention debulking surgery. Reprinted with permission from van der Burg et al. N Engl J Med 1995; **332**: 629–34. Copyright © 1995 Massachusetts Medical Society. All rights reserved

Recurrent disease

Surgery for recurrent disease has a limited role in the treatment of women in whom the tumour recurs late (more than 12 months after chemotherapy) and in whom the intention is to treat with further chemotherapy, but this would be a good subject for a randomized trial.

Conclusion

The role of surgery in ovarian cancer is to make the diagnosis. It will cure many patients with borderline disease and early-stage ovarian cancer. It will relieve the symptoms in many women with advanced tumours, but in this context in should be seen as an adjunct to chemotherapy and not an end in itself.

References

1. Morice P, Camatte S, El Hassan J *et al.* Clinical outcomes and fertility after conservative treatment of ovarian borderline tumours. *Fertil Steril* 2001; **75**: 92–6.

2. Zanetta G, Rota S, Chiari S *et al.* Behaviour of borderline ovarian tumours with particular interest to persistence, recurrence, and progression to invasive carcinoma: a prospective study. *J Clin Oncol* 2001; **19**: 2658–64.

3. Vergote I, De Brabanter J, Fyles A *et al.* Prognostic importance of degree of differentiation and cyst rupture in stage I invasive epithelial ovarian carcinoma. *Lancet* 2001; **357**: 176–82.

4. Griffiths CT, Parker LM, Fuller AF. Role of cytoreductive surgical treatment in the management of advanced ovarian cancer. *Cancer Treat Rep* 1979; **63**: 235–40.

5. Hunter RW, Alexander ND, Soutter WP. Meta-analysis of surgery in advanced ovarian carcinoma: is maximum cytoreductive surgery an independent determinant of prognosis? *Am J Obstet Gynecol* 1992; **166**: 504–11.

6. van der Burg ME, van Lent M, Buyse M *et al.* The effect of debulking surgery after induction chemotherapy on the prognosis in advanced epithelial ovarian cancer. *N Engl J Med* 1995; **332**: 629–34.

Pathology and its prognostic importance

Michael Wells, University of Sheffield Medical School, Sheffield

Histogenesis

There are several different histological types of ovarian epithelial neoplasia. One of the common themes, particularly if we consider serous tumours as the paradigm of epithelial ovarian neoplasia, is origin from mesothelium. The mesothelium lines the peritoneal cavity and covers the surface of the ovary, and has the propensity to undergo Müllerian metaplasia. It is hypothesized that the surface epithelium of the ovary undergoes ovulatory trauma in response to ovulation, resulting in epithelial clefts or invaginations (Figure 1). These invaginations may then undergo cystic change to form ovarian epithelial inclusion cysts (Figure 2). It has been shown that these cysts are increased in 'normal' ovaries adjacent to carcinoma.[1]

The incidental finding of pre-invasive neoplastic change is rare in otherwise macroscopically unremarkable ovaries. However, such changes are seen in the surface epithelium adjacent to carcinoma. It has been shown that such ovarian intraepithelial neoplasia exhibits overexpression of p53 protein, which in some cases is a manifestation of *p53* mutation.[2] However, there are other explanations for p53 overexpression, such as binding to MDM2.

Figure 3 shows ovarian intraepithelial neoplasia with dysplasia of the epithelium lining an inclusion cyst, nuclear pleomorphism, increased mitotic activity and increased expression of p53 protein.

Histological findings

Recent work on ovaries removed at prophylactic oophorectomy from women with a high familial risk of ovarian cancer has been disappointing. If ovarian intraepithelial neoplasia (ie precancer of the ovary) exists as a distinct lesion, then it is in such ovaries that we would expect to find it. However, microscopic cancers have been reported only rarely, and most studies report no distinctive features compared with control ovaries.[3] The one exception to this was a paper by Salazar and colleagues,[4] in which deep cortical clefts, surface papillomas and fine-surface papillations were reported. No other group has been able to repeat this work, and it was an unblinded study.

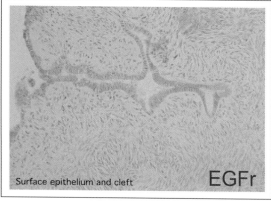

Surface epithelium and cleft — EGFr

Figure 1: Ovarian surface epithelium extending into a cortical cleft showing epidermal growth factor receptor expression.

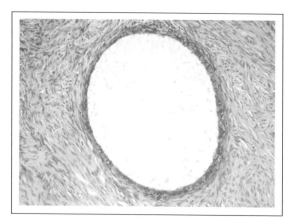

Figure 2: A benign ovarian cortical epithelial inclusion cyst.

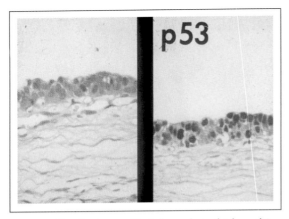

Figure 3: Ovarian intraepithelial neoplasia (high grade) or severe epithelial dysplasia showing intense p53 *protein expression which may equate with* p53 *mutation.*

Epithelial tumour types

The classification of ovarian neoplasia is complex.[5] Epithelial tumours, which are only one of four major tumour types in the ovary, can be divided into five broad groups (listed below in order of frequency), each of which may be benign, borderline or malignant:

- serous
- endometrioid
- mucinous
- clear-cell
- transitional-cell.

Clear-cell tumours are arguably a variant of endometrioid tumours and show an association with endometriosis. This paper will not discuss the rare small-cell carcinoma of the ovary, a tumour with a poor prognosis seen in young women, because its histogenesis remains uncertain.

Serous tumours

Table 1 compares the most common genetic abnormalities of serous borderline tumours and serous carcinomas; the genotype of these two tumour types is quite different. Although borderline tumours show some of the features that we associate with malignancy, they lack the most important feature – stromal invasion. It is tempting to believe that the majority of serous-type carcinomas of the ovary arise from a pre-existing borderline tumour, however, there is no evidence for this. Rather, borderline tumours are distinct entities that attain a phase of phenotypic stability and, with rare exceptions, are not associated with invasion in the primary tumour.

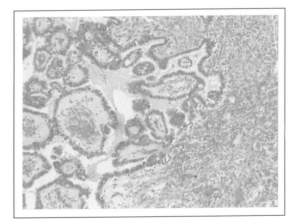

Figure 4: Borderline serous tumour.

Figure 4 shows a serous borderline tumour. Although the epithelium has a papillary appearance, there is a relatively well-defined interface between the epithelium and the underlying stroma. The long-term survival of patients with serous borderline tumours confined to the ovaries exceeds 99%.[6] It is when serous borderline tumours are associated with peritoneal lesions that difficulties arise. Four types of peritoneal lesion may occur in patients with serous borderline tumours:

Table 1 Comparison of serous borderline tumours and serous carcinomas

	Borderline	Carcinoma
p53 mutation	Absent	Frequent
Loss of heterozygosity	Long arm of the inactivated x chromosome	Multiple chromosomes (1, 6q, 11, 13q, 17p, 17q)
Microsatellite instability	Present	Absent
KRAS & BRAF mutation	Present	Absent

- endosalpingiosis
- borderline lesions
- desmoplastic, non-invasive lesions
- invasive lesions.

Endosalpingiosis is a benign condition that is a common incidental finding in the peritoneal cavity. It can be thought of as the tubal equivalent of endometriosis and simply reflects the capacity of the peritoneal mesothelium to undergo Müllerian metaplasia. Figure 5 shows a peritoneal or implant lesion that is designated borderline because it shows cytological atypia. Figure 6 shows abnormal epithelium with a tripolar mitosis and is an invasive implant within the peritoneal cavity.

Patients with serous borderline tumours who do badly tend to have invasive peritoneal implants, whereas the five- to ten-year survival for patients with non-invasive implants approaches 100%.

This has led to a further analysis of the primary tumours associated with invasive disease. Kurman and colleagues suggested that the majority of borderline tumours associated with invasive implants in the peritoneum show a typical micropapillary pattern, as shown in Figure 7.[8] Kurman believes that these should be called 'micropapillary serous carcinomas' despite the fact that there is no invasion of the primary tumour. These micropapillary lesions are well-differentiated and non-invasive, show strong association with invasive implants and recur frequently as invasive carcinomas. Kurman reports that they have a 10-year survival of 60%.[7-10] However, this work remains controversial, and whilst reference will be made to micropapillary serous carcinoma in the forthcoming World Health Organization 'Blue Book' (*Tumours of the breast and female genital tract*), it has not been accepted as a distinct pathological entity.

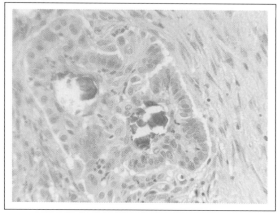

Figure 5: A non-invasive borderline peritoneal implant showing histological appearances similar to the primary ovarian serous borderline tumour.

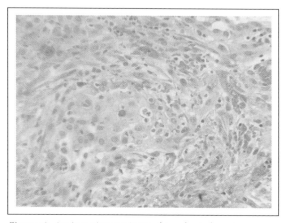

Figure 6: An invasive peritoneal implant showing cytological atypia, an abnormal mitotic figure and a stromal desmoplastic response.

Mucinous borderline tumours

In the context of mucinous borderline tumours, the lesion that has been most often associated with a poor prognosis is pseudomyxoma peritonei. However, it is now clear that most cases of apparent mucinous borderline tumours of the ovary associated with pseudomyxoma peritonei are not primary ovarian tumours but represent very well-differentiated metastases from a primary appendiceal tumour.[11, 12] Therefore, meticulous examination of the large intestine in general and the appendix in particular is of crucial importance if a mucinous tumour is suspected. If we remove those mucinous tumours with a poor prognosis and appreciate that they are not primary ovarian tumours at all, then the overall prognosis for mucinous borderline tumours of the ovary is excellent.

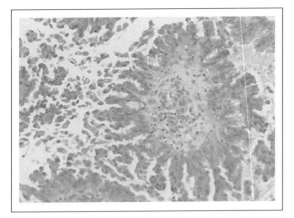

Figure 7: A 'micropapillary serous carcinoma'; the variant of serous borderline tumour considered by Kurman to be particularly associated with invasive peritoneal disease and a poor prognosis.

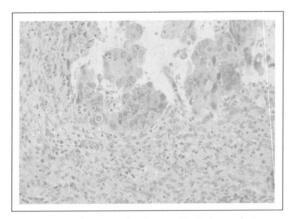

Figure 8: Atypia or ovarian intraepithelial neoplasia within the epithelial lining of an endometriotic cyst. Note the typical endometrial-type stroma.

Endometriosis and ovarian cancer

A lot of interesting work has been carried out on the role of endometriosis and its relationship to ovarian carcinoma.[13] Although it would be alarmist to state that endometriosis is a premalignant condition, it is clear that it does have neoplastic potential. Recent work has shown that endometriosis is monoclonal,[14] and that loss of heterozygosity is seen in 75% of cases associated with endometrioid adenocarcinoma when the associated endometriosis is microdissected and subjected to molecular analysis.[15, 16] However, Campbell and colleagues have also shown that there is loss of heterozygosity in 28% of cases of endometriosis even without associated carcinoma.

Figure 8 shows ovarian intraepithelial neoplasia occurring within endometriosis.

Prognostic factors

Prognostic factors for ovarian cancer include six main parameters:

- stage
- histological type
- histological grading
- ploidy
- morphometric indices
- oncogenes and tumour suppressor genes.

There is no substitute in the assessment of ovarian tumours for the meticulous examination of the haematoxylin and eosin-stained section.

This paper will not discuss stage, because that looks at ovarian cancer from a clinical rather than a pathological point of view. Space limitations also prevent us from discussing morphometric indices.

Histological type

There is some evidence that the histological type has an influence on prognosis. It has been suggested that endometrioid tumours when combined with foci of serous adenocarcinoma have a poorer prognosis.[17] Mucinous carcinoma at an advanced stage may have a poorer prognosis as such tumours are thought to be more resistant to platinum therapy.[18] There is also evidence to show that clear-cell cancer, particularly in stage I disease, has a poorer prognosis;[11] there may well be a case for the institution of chemotherapy for clear-cell carcinoma even in stage I disease, but this remains controversial.

Histological grading

There is no universally accepted grading system for ovarian cancer and there is considerable inter- and intra-observer variation. I believe that it would be better to use the terms 'low-grade' and 'high-grade' tumours rather than using the three-tier classification of well, moderately and poorly differentiated tumours. We do not conventionally grade clear-cell carcinoma because we regard it as a high-grade tumour.

A more refined grading system analogous to the Nottingham Prognostic Index used in breast carcinoma has recently been proposed.[19] This combines architectural features, nuclear grade and mitotic count. However, ovarian cancer is much more heterogeneous than breast carcinoma, and it remains to be seen whether this work is reproducible. It is important to remember that even if we use the term 'cancer' as meaning an epithelial tumour, then ovarian cancer is not a single entity.

Ploidy

Ploidy refers to the DNA content of the cells. Aneuploid tumours have irregular amounts of DNA within the cells. We know that 45% of Stage I ovarian tumours are aneuploid and the evidence suggests that aneuploidy is an independent adverse prognostic factor.[20] There may be a case for carrying out ploidy analysis in Stage I ovarian carcinoma to select those patients who can be treated conservatively.

Work done on borderline tumours has shown that more than 90% are diploid.[20] However, a proportion of borderline tumours are aneuploid, and it has been suggested that this is an independent indicator of poor prognosis. Moreover, we know that diploid primary tumours may be associated with aneuploid peritoneal lesions, so there is a case for carrying out ploidy analysis on peritoneal lesions.[20] The demonstration of diploidy in a non-invasive peritoneal implant may provide further reassurance that the patient can be managed conservatively.

Oncogenes and tumour suppressor genes

Three major genes have been implicated in sporadic ovarian cancer: *p53*, *c-myc* and *c-erbB-2*. However, the evidence for the roles of mutation, amplification and protein overexpression of these genes is conflicting. Currently, there is no place for the testing of these genes in routine diagnostic practice to determine the prognosis of patients with ovarian cancer.[20]

Conclusion

Ovarian epithelial neoplasia is histologically diverse and a clear distinction must be drawn between borderline and invasive disease. Molecular pathology has done much to improve our understanding of the pathogenesis of epithelial neoplasia and different molecular pathways are being elucidated relating to the predominant histological types of serous, endometrioid and mucinous tumours. However, for the day-to-day diagnosis and management of ovarian tumours, there is no substitute for careful histological interpretation, which can also provide useful insight into the prognosis of an individual tumour. Ancillary techniques (such as ploidy) determination have a limited role.

References

1. Feeley KM, Wells M. Precursor lesions of ovarian epithelial malignancy. *Histopathology* 2001; **38**: 87–95.

2. Hutson R, Ramsdale A, Wells M. p53 protein expression in putative precursor lesions of epithelial ovarian cancer. *Histopathology* 1995; **27**: 367–71.

3. Werness BA, Eltabbakh GH. Familial ovarian cancer and early ovarian cancer: biologic, pathologic, and clinical features. *Int J Gynecol Pathol* 2001; **20**: 48–63.

4. Salazar H, Godwin AK, Daly MB *et al*. Microscopic benign and malignant neoplasms and a cancer-prone phenotype in prophylactic oophorectomies. *J Natl Cancer Inst* 1996; **88**: 1810–20.

5. Fox H, Wells M. Ovarian tumours: classification, histogenesis and aetiology. In: Haines & Taylor, *Obstetrical and Gynaecological Pathology Fifth Edition*, 2003: 693–712.

6. Fox H. Ovarian tumours of borderline malignancy: time for a reappraisal? *Curr Diag Pathol* 1996; **78**: 111–34.

7. Burks RT, Sherman ME, Kurman RJ. Micropapillary serous carcinoma of the ovary. A distinctive low-grade carcinoma related to serous borderline tumours. *Am J Surg Pathol* 1996; **20**: 1319–30.

8. Bell KA, Smith Sehdev AE, Kurman RJ. Refined diagnostic criteria for implants associated with ovarian atypical proliferative serous tumours (borderline) and micropapillary serous carcinomas. *Am J Surg Pathol* 2001; **25**: 419–32.

9. Singer G, Kurman RJ, Chang HW *et al*. Diverse tumorigenic pathways in ovarian serous carcinoma. *Am J Pathol* 2002; **160**: 1223–8.

10. Singer G, Shih IeM, Truskinovsky A *et al*. Mutational Analysis of K-ras Segregates Ovarian Carcinomas into Two Types: Invasive MPSC (Low-grade Tumor) and Conventional Serous Carcinoma (High-grade Tumor). *Int J Gynecol Pathol* 2003; **22**: 37–41.

11. Fox H, Wells M. Surface epithleial tumours of the ovary. In: Haines & Taylor, *Obstetrical and Gynaecological Pathology Fifth Edition*, 2003: 713–43.

12. Ronnett BM, Shmookler BM, Diener-West M *et al*. Immunohistochemical evidence supporting the appendiceal origin of pseudomyxoma peritonei. *Int J Gynecol Pathol* 1997; **16**: 1–9.

13. Fukunaga M, Nomura K, Ishikawa E, Ushigome S. Ovarian atypical endometriosis: its close association with malignant epithelial tumours. *Histopathology* 1997; **30**: 249–55.

14. Tamura M, Fukaya T, Murakami *et al*. Analysis of clonality in human endometriotic cysts based on evaluation of X-chromsome inactivation in archival formalin-fixed, paraffin-embedded tissue. *Lab Invest* 1998; **78**: 213–18.

15. Jiang X, Hitchcock A, Bryan EJ *et al*. Microsatellite analysis of endometriosis reveals loss of heterozygosity at candidate ovarian tumour suppressor gene loci. *Cancer Res* 1996; **56**: 3534–9.

16. Jiang X, Morland SJ, Hitchcock A *et al*. Allelotyping of endometriosis with adjacent ovarian carcinoma reveals evidence of a common lineage. *Cancer Res* 1998; **58**: 1707–12.

17. Tornos C, Silva EG, Khorana SM, Burke TW. High-stage endometrioid carcinoma of the ovary. Prognostic significance of pure versus mixed histologic types. *Am J Surg Pathol* 1994; **18**: 687–93.

18. Omura GA, Brady MF, Homesley HD *et al*. Long-term follow-up and prognostic factor analysis in advanced ovarian cancer: the Gynecologic Oncology Group experience. *J Clin Oncol* 1991; **9**: 1138–50.

19. Silverberg SG. Histopathologic grading of ovarian carcinoma: a review and proposal. *Int J Gynecol Pathol* 2000; **19**: 7–15.

20. Cheung ANY, Fox H, Wells M. The application of new techniques in gynaecological pathology. In: Haines & Taylor, *Obstetrical and Gynaecological Pathology Fifth Edition* 2003: 1595–626.

First-line chemotherapy

Stanley Kaye, Royal Marsden Hospital, London

Chemotherapy has a role both in the adjuvant treatment of stage I ovarian cancer and in the optimal primary treatment of women with advanced ovarian cancer. This paper will cover both topics.

Stage I ovarian cancer

The results of two large studies running over nine years were pooled to determine whether platinum-based chemotherapy is better than simply watching patients with stage I ovarian cancer. The first International Collaborative Ovarian Neoplasm (ICON-1) study in the UK was based on the uncertainty principle, while the European Adjuvant Chemotherapy in Ovarian Neoplasm (ACTION) study involved a slightly better defined group of early ovarian cancer patients. Patients were randomized to receive no treatment or to receive platinum chemotherapy (single-agent carboplatin or combination including paclitaxel) and then followed up for a median of three years. Overall the studies showed a significant benefit for chemotherapy in both recurrence-free survival and overall survival.[1]

These results received some criticism, based mainly around the potential inadequacy of staging. One view was that the patients were not staged adequately and that some patients may well have had undiagnosed stage III rather than early disease. Subgroup analysis showed no clear evidence for this, although it remains a possibility. Nevertheless, the pragmatic view is that the studies took place in the framework of contemporary clinical practice and the conclusions were clear.

I believe that in women with stage I ovarian cancer where there is a concern about the possibility of relapse – ie not well-differentiated stage Ia ovarian cancers, for which the outlook is excellent – then it makes sense to give chemotherapy.

Advanced ovarian cancer

The majority of patients with advanced disease now receive chemotherapy, which is usually platinum-based. The response rate to chemotherapy is very high, and it clearly prolongs survival. Unfortunately, although some patients (probably those with well-differentiated tumours) are alive and disease-free 10 years later, most patients relapse within one to three years.

Historical perspective

Platinum was introduced in the 1970s, and cisplatin quickly became established as part of the treatment of ovarian cancer. Paclitaxel was tested in the mid-1990s in randomized trials. The Gynecologic Oncology Group 111 (GOG-111) study demonstrated that the addition of paclitaxel to cisplatin was superior to the then standard therapy of cyclophosphamide and cisplatin;[2] the key difference being an overall survival benefit of one year. Another study showed the same results in patients not only with bulky disease, but also with minimal residual disease.[3] In 1998, paclitaxel/cisplatin became the gold-standard treatment of advanced ovarian cancer.

At about the same time, the Medical Research Council (MRC) looked at all the randomized trials that had tried to determine whether there was any difference between cisplatin and carboplatin. It was widely believed that carboplatin could not be as effective as cisplatin since it was better tolerated, and it was thought that toxicity equated with better efficacy. However, the MRC overview essentially showed no difference between the two drugs, even in patients with low-volume residual disease.[4] The next question was whether carboplatin could be used with paclitaxel. Three studies addressed this, comparing standard cisplatin/paclitaxel versus carboplatin/paclitaxel. These studies showed no sign of any detriment when using carboplatin; in fact, there was a (statistically non-significant) benefit for the carboplatin arm in one of the trials.[5] Based on this, many oncologists have concluded that standard therapy should comprise paclitaxel and carboplatin.

Improving the results

Although the results with paclitaxel/carboplatin have been encouraging, we still need to do better. Various trials have looked at maintenance treatment with paclitaxel, the addition of other cytotoxic drugs, sequential treatment regimes, alternative taxanes, high-dose/intraperitoneal therapy and radio-immunotherapy.

Maintenance treatment

Studies to determine whether further chemotherapy with cisplatin or carboplatin might prevent relapse following initial response (radiologically or according to CA125 level) were essentially negative. Until recently, most oncologists were therefore sceptical about the value of maintenance chemotherapy. This has somewhat changed as a result of a study from the USA which looked at continuing treatment with paclitaxel in patients who had initial treatment.[6] Women were randomized after initial treatment to receive paclitaxel for either three or 12 more months. The study was closed after a total of 262 patients had been randomized because an interim analysis showed that there were significantly more recurrences in the three-month arm. While there was therefore a significant difference in progression-free survival that favoured the longer treatment, there was no overall difference in survival. This study has caused considerable controversy (chiefly because of its small size), but in the USA a number of oncologists now believe that standard treatment should include continuing treatment with paclitaxel.

Addition of other cytotoxics and sequential treatment regimes

Several new drugs are available that could be incorporated into the first-line treatment of ovarian cancer, including epirubicin, gemcitabine, topotecan, irinotecan and doxil. There are three ways of doing this:

- add another drug to the conventional combination
- use a sequential doublet
- use a different sequential regime.

The most mature data are for epirubicin: two studies investigated whether paclitaxel/epirubicin/carboplatin is better than paclitaxel/carboplatin.[7, 8] Interestingly, both studies have demonstrated a slight benefit and a combined analysis may demonstrate a clear survival difference. However, unsurprisingly, there is more toxicity with the three-drug combination, so we need to investigate other ways of adding epirubicin. The use of a sequential doublet is part of an ongoing international four-arm study in which the new agents being assessed are gemcitabine, topotecan and doxil. Another study is looking at sequencing in which the third drug (topotecan) is given after paclitaxel/carboplatin.

A major issue is how we should interpret the results of the GOG-132[9] and the ICON-3 trials,[10] both of which reported that there was no benefit for adding paclitaxel to platinum. Why is it that two drugs that are clearly effective individually are not better than one, when this is not what we see in most other cancers? One reason could be that there was an early crossover in the GOG-132 study, but this probably did not account for the whole difference. There is also the possibility that the two drugs are antagonistic when given together, and there are some experimental data to support this. The Scottish Gynaecological Cancer Trials Group is currently investigating whether a novel sequential approach might minimize any potential antagonism which may exist when giving paclitaxel and carboplatin in combination.[11] In separate feasibility studies, patients receive four courses of single agent carboplatin (AUC 7) followed by weekly or three-weekly paclitaxel or docetaxel, together with gemcitabine or irinotecan.

There are some molecular reasons for thinking that giving initial treatment as a full dose of a single agent may take advantage of the fact that ovarian cancer cells, according to their *p53* status, have different response rates to platinum and paclitaxel, and that addressing these separately might make sense. This dosing is well tolerated.

At the Royal Marsden Hospital, we do not consider single-agent carboplatin to be standard first-line therapy and will frequently recommend the paclitaxel/carboplatin regimen. However, overall the data indicate a rather modest benefit for the combination and therefore it is important to discuss the facts with patients when recommending which treatment to choose. The current National Institute for Clinical Excellence (NICE) guidelines recommend both the combination and the single agent for first-line treatment.

Alternative taxanes

A possible alternative to paclitaxel might be docetaxel and many oncologists believe that in other diseases, particularly breast cancer, docetaxel is more effective. A phase II study has shown that docetaxel is active in paclitaxel-resistant ovarian cancer.[12] Early studies suggested that it was less neurotoxic in combination with carboplatin. In the Scottish Randomized Trial in Ovarian Cancer (SCOTROC) study,[13] over 1000 patients received either paclitaxel/carboplatin or docetaxel/carboplatin. The results so far have shown equivalence between the two in terms of response rate and survival. There was significantly less neurotoxicity on the docetaxel arm but significantly more neutropenia than with paclitaxel. Many oncologists have concluded that while efficacy seems to be the same, the toxicity profile indicates that docetaxel is a valid alternative to paclitaxel, particularly for patients in whom the possibility of neurotoxicity may be especially problematic. Scalp cooling to avoid hair loss is also a feasible option with docetaxel, so it may be worth discussing this with the patient.

Molecularly targeted agents

There has been a large increase in interest in novel agents which target specific signalling pathways in tumour cells and offer the possibility of specific tumour growth inhibition. One such pathway, which is certainly relevant to ovarian cancer, is the epidermal growth factor (EGF) receptor pathway. This pathway can be disrupted clinically by monoclonal antibodies or small molecule tyrosine kinase inhibitors (eg Iressa, Tarceva). There is evidence from a phase II trial of clinical activity in refractory ovarian cancer for Tarceva,[14] and preclinical evidence indicating a greater than additive effect when these agents are added to chemotherapy in human tumour xenografts. The challenge for the future is how to incorporate these novel agents in to first-line treatment; initial experience in lung cancer indicates that this is not straightforward and careful patient selection may ultimately be required.

High-dose/intraperitoneal chemotherapy

There has been a considerable interest in treating ovarian cancer with higher doses of chemotherapy, either systemically or intraperitoneally. However, only one randomized trial of high-dose chemotherapy has been completed. In this trial it was given as a consolidation treatment and compared with conventional-dose chemotherapy. The study did show a survival benefit,[15] but accrual took several years to complete. I believe that the high-dose approach needs to be studied properly, but it probably will not be widely applicable.

An alternative approach is to put the drug in contact with the tumour cells to get the highest exposure, ie by giving it intraperitoneally. There have been three positive studies of first-line intraperitoneal chemotherapy.[16-18] However, two of these were flawed in trial design mainly because of differences in drug dose. We still cannot draw any firm conclusions about intraperitoneal chemotherapy but it remains an important area for ongoing research.

Radio-immunotherapy and immunotherapy

Another approach to regional treatment is to deliver therapeutic doses of ionizing radiation in to the peritoneal cavity.[19] This is best achieved by linking the radionuclide to an antibody which will localize on tumour cells. Non-randomized trials (involving yttrium and the MUC-1 antigen) indicate the promise of this treatment and randomized studies are ongoing.

Another immunotherapy approach has been studied in one trial that added gamma-interferon subcutaneously to first-line chemotherapy.[20] This showed a significant survival benefit, and although the mechanism of action is unclear further studies are now looking at interferon with larger patient numbers.

Conclusion

The outstanding issues in first-line ovarian cancer chemotherapy are:

- to determine whether new combinations and/or sequences prove superior both to paclitaxel/carboplatin and to single-agent carboplatin
- whether some form of maintenance treatment could be useful
- how to assess the potential additional benefit of novel molecularly targeted agents.

In addition, if we could understand, from the point of view of translational research, what causes acquired drug resistance in tumours during chemotherapy, we could begin large-scale rational trials of reversal using agents, several of which are already undergoing preliminary clinical assessment.

References

1. Trimbos JB, Parmar M, Vergote I *et al*. International Collaborative Ovarian Neoplasm trial 1 and Adjuvant ChemoTherapy In Ovarian Neoplasm trial: two parallel randomized phase III trials of adjuvant chemotherapy in patients with early-stage ovarian carcinoma. *J Natl Cancer Inst* 2003; **95**: 105–12.

2. McGuire WP, Hoskins WJ, Brady MF *et al*. Cyclophosphamide and cisplatin compared with paclitaxel and cisplatin in patients with stage III and stage IV ovarian cancer. *N Engl J Med* 1996; **334**: 1–6.

3. Piccart MJ, Bertelsen K, James K *et al*. Randomized intergroup trial of cisplatin-paclitaxel versus cisplatin-cyclophosphamide in women with advanced epithelial ovarian cancer: three-year results. *J Natl Cancer Inst* 2000; **92**: 699–708.

4. Aabo K, Adams M, Adnitt P *et al*. Chemotherapy in advanced ovarian cancer: four systematic meta-analyses of individual patient data from 37 randomized trials. Advanced Ovarian Cancer Trialists' Group. *Br J Cancer* 1998; **78**: 1479–87.

5. Ozols RF. Update on the management of ovarian cancer. *Cancer J* 2002; **8 (Suppl 1)**: S22–S30.

6. Ozols RF. Future directions in the treatment of ovarian cancer. *Semin Oncol* 2002; **29 (Suppl 1)**: 32–42.

7. Weber B, Kuha W, Goupil A *et al*. Epirubicin/paclitaxel/carboplatin vs. paclitaxel/carboplatin in first line treatment of ovarian cancer – prelim result. A GINECO randomized trial. *Europ J Cancer* 2001; **37 (Suppl 6)**: 1018 (abst).

8. Kristensen G, Vergste I, Stuart G *et al*. First-line treatment of Stage III-IV ovarian cancer with paclitaxel/epirubicin/carboplatin versus paclitaxel/carboplatin: interim results of an Intergroup trial *Proc ASCO* 2002; **21**: 805 (abst).

9. Muggia FM, Braly PS, Brady MF *et al*. Phase III randomized study of cisplatin versus paclitaxel versus cisplatin and paclitaxel in patients with suboptimal stage III or IV ovarian cancer: a gynecologic oncology group study. *J Clin Oncol* 2000; **18**: 106–15.

10. Paclitaxel plus carboplatin versus standard chemotherapy with either single-agent carboplatin or cyclophosphamide, doxorubicin, and cisplatin in women with ovarian cancer: the ICON3 randomised trial. *Lancet* 2002; **360**: 505–15.

11. Rustin G, Atkinson R, Osborne R *et al*. Preliminary results of SCOTROC-2A a feasibility study of

carboplatin then sequential docetaxel, or 2 schedules of docetaxel-gemcitabine. *Proc ASCO* 2002; **21**: 810 (abst).

12. Verschraegen C, Sittisomwong T, Kudelka AP *et al*. Docetaxel for patients with paclitaxel-resistant Mullerian carcinoma. *J Clin Oncol* 2000; **18**: 2733–9.

13. Vasey PA. Survival and long-term toxicity results of the SCOTROC study, docetaxel-carboplatin versus paclitaxel-carboplatin in advanced ovarian cancer. *Proc ASCO* 2002; **21**: 804 (abst).

14. Finkler N, Gordon A, Crozier M *et al*. Phase 2 evaluation of OSI-774, a potent oral antagonist of the EGFR-TK in patients with advanced ovarian carcinoma. *Proc ASCO* 2001; **20**: 831 (abst).

15. Cure H, Battista C, Gustalla J *et al*. Phase III randomized trial of high dose chemotherapy and PBSC support as consolidation in patients with responsive low burden advanced ovarian cancer: preliminary results of a GINECO/FNLCC/SFGM-TC study. *Proc ASCO* 2001; **20**: 204a.

16. Armstrong DK, Bundy BN, Baergen R *et al*. Randomized phase III study of intravenous (IV) paclitaxel and cisplatin versus IV paclitaxel, intraperitoneal (IP) cisplatin and IP paclitaxel in optimal stage III epithelial ovarian cancer: a Gynecologic Oncology Group trial (GOC 172). *Proc ASCO* 2002; **21**: 803 (abst).

17. Alberts DS, Liu PY, Hannigan EV *et al*. Intraperitoneal cisplatin plus intravenous cyclophosphamide versus intravenous cisplatin plus intravenous cyclophosphamide for stage III ovarian cancer. *N Engl J Med* 1996; **335**: 1950–5.

18. Markman M, Bundy BN, Alberts DS *et al*. Phase III trial of standard-dose intravenous cisplatin plus paclitaxel versus moderately high-dose carboplatin followed by intravenous paclitaxel and intraperitoneal cisplatin in small-volume stage III ovarian cancer carcinoma: an intergroup study of the Gynecologic Oncology Group, Southwestern Oncology Group and Eastern Cooperative Oncology Group. *J Clin Oncol* 2001; **19**: 1001–7.

19. Nicholson S, Gooden CS, Hird V *et al*. Radioimmunotherapy after chemotherapy compared to chemotherapy alone in the treatment of advanced ovarian cancer: a matched analysis. *Oncol Rep* 1998; **5**: 223–6.

20. Windbichler GH, Hausmaninger H, Stummvoll W *et al*. Interferon-gamma in the first-line therapy of ovarian cancer: a randomized phase III trial. *Br J Cancer* 2000; **82**: 1138–44.

Relapse chemotherapy and the role of tumour markers

Gordon Rustin, Mount Vernon Hospital, Northwood, Middlesex

The main aim of management after initial therapy is to maintain quality of life. This involves considering the whole concept of how we will deal with the patient after initial treatment. We also have to appreciate the role of follow-up, but we can do this only if we appreciate the role of relapse therapy. Relapse therapy is palliative therapy: we cannot cure a patient with ovarian cancer once they have relapsed. Therefore, we have to think very carefully about why we follow these patients. As we do not know whether early diagnosis of relapse makes any difference to survival, we may only be inducing anxiety in our patients.

The great majority of ovarian cancer relapses are picked up on history alone, without examining the patient. Unlike in endometrial/cervical cancer, for example, where local relapses are potentially curable, follow-up internal examinations in ovarian cancer have little impact other than to worry the patient.

Follow-up CA125 testing

We know that follow-up CA125 testing can diagnose relapse early on. A definition based on doubling CA125 levels from the upper limit of normal or from a nadir level is being increasingly used in clinical trials.[1] Once relapse has been diagnosed, there is then a temptation to give earlier treatment. This may prolong survival and delay the requirement for in-patient care, eg for removal of ascites, intestinal obstruction or pain control. Doing a CA125 test might also avoid radiological examinations.

However, the main reason for carrying out CA125 testing is to give reassurance. I believe that this is wrong, because about half the patients with small-volume disease will have a normal CA125 level, thus giving them false hope. Of course, it is easy to concede to patient pressure and do the blood test; it takes a lot longer to counsel the patient and explain the reasons for not doing the test. Measuring CA125 during follow-up may also increase anxiety, inducing a disease known as 'CA125 psychosis'.

If the CA125 level goes up, the patient 'knows' that she has relapsed and is going to die. There will then, of course, be huge pressure to restart therapy, even if the patient is asymptomatic. It is difficult to persuade a patient with a raised CA125 level that there is no evidence that early retreatment helps.

A large ongoing trial organized by the Medical Research Council (MRC) and European Organization for Research and Treatment of Cancer (EORTC) is studying the value of follow-up CA125 testing. Patients in complete clinical remission after initial treatment have regular CA125 tests, the results of which are made available only to the MRC; this makes clinic attendances far more relaxed because no CA125 psychosis is involved. If the CA125 level rises, patients are randomized between (a) the clinician being informed and giving retreatment within one month or (b) the clinician not being informed and only retreating when signs or symptoms indicate relapse.

I believe that we should discourage regular CA125 follow-up unless patients are in the MRC/EORTC trial. We should be counselling our patients about the possible advantages and disadvantages of CA125 testing. A good compromise in patients not in this trial is to give them a CA125 request form and advise them to get the blood test done only if they've got symptoms of relapse.

Prediction of response to subsequent chemotherapy

It has been known for several years that a patient who relapses more than six months after platinum therapy has a very high chance of responding to further platinum therapy.[2] A large Canadian study looked at the factors that determine whether a patient will respond to subsequent chemotherapy. Univariate analysis indicated that serous histology, tumour size less than 5 cm, normal haemoglobin level and a treatment-free interval of more than six months predicted a good response to subsequent chemotherapy.[3] On multivariate analysis, serous histology, number of disease sites and smaller tumour size were found to be good predictors of response.[3]

The important thing that this study showed is that we should not wait until a patient is very ill before trying relapse therapy. This suggests that a follow-up system in which the patient can telephone a nurse to discuss her symptoms rather than waiting for the next hospital appointment may have advantages.

Treatment for relapsed ovarian cancer

Once a patient has relapsed, there are various options. The first thing one should always consider is whether to repeat the initial therapy or not. Surgery may be used to remove tumour masses in patients who have survived for a number of years and who have slow-growing disease. Occasionally, radiotherapy is used for symptomatic control of vaginal bleeding and pelvic pain. There are also a number of chemotherapeutic approaches.[4]

Early relapse

Patients with early relapse (within six months of initial treatment) have a worse prognosis than those who relapse later. Table 1, which is used by a large sample of oncologists in this country, shows the current standard treatments for early-relapsed ovarian cancer in the UK. The only chemotherapy regimen that has been reported to have a response rate greater than 40% in early relapsed ovarian cancer is weekly cisplatin plus oral etoposide.[5,6] We use cisplatin rather than carboplatin in this regimen because carboplatin is too myelosuppressive to be given weekly unless the dose is reduced considerably. Interestingly, the National Institute for Clinical Excellence (NICE)-approved drugs for early relapse disease – paclitaxel, topotecan and liposomal doxorubicin – have response rates of less than 15% in this situation, so this needs to be studied further.

A tolerability study comparing liposomal doxorubicin with topotecan showed that topotecan causes far worse leucopenia, thrombocytopenia and anaemia (Figure 1). Although this myelosupression appears severe, it rarely leads to major clinical problems. However, liposomal doxorubicin can cause plantar-palmar erythema, which may lead to severe desquamation of the skin if treatment is continued – this does not occur with topotecan. Most clinicians, of course, look at the profile shown in Figure 1 and give liposomal doxorubicin because it appears to be better tolerated. Liposomal doxorubicin also has the advantage of being given as a single short injection every four weeks whilst topotecan has to be given as five injections daily for five days every three weeks.

Table 1 Current standard treatments in the UK for early relapse of ovarian cancer (replies to questionnaires from 57 clinicians in 47 centres). As some clinicians listed more than one treatment, the total is greater than 100%.

Treatment	Percentage
Liposomal doxorubicin	51
Etoposide±cisplatin	33
Topotecan	32
Paclitaxel (if not given first-line)	14
Chlorambucil	4
Epirubicin/cisplatin/5FU	4
New drug studies/in-house trials	4
TCA-ovary study	4
Warfarin, cyclophosphamide and tamoxifen	2
Gemcitabine/carboplatin	2
Gemcitabine/treosulfan	2
Mitoxantrone/paclitaxel	2
Tamoxifen	2

TCA, tumour chemosensitivity assay

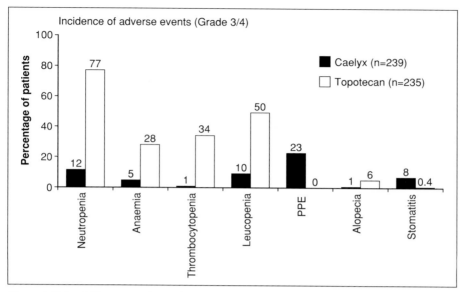

Figure 1: Tolerability comparison of topotecan and liposomal doxorubicin.
Gordon et al. J Clin Oncol 2001; **19**: 3312–22. Reprinted with permission from the American Society of Clinical Oncology

Late relapse

In patients who relapse after more than six months, the standard chemotherapy regimes all have response rates in excess of 20%, even reaching 60% in long-interval patients. Many oncologists consider repeating the initial therapy. The results of the fourth International Collaborative Ovarian Neoplasm (ICON-4) study suggest that using paclitaxel at this point offers a significant advantage in terms of time to progression and 2-year mortality rate when compared to non-paclitaxel platinum regimens, even in patients who have previously received paclitaxel as first-line therapy. These results will appear in the proceedings of ASCO in May 2003.

There are also other drugs that we should consider. Many patients do not want to lose their hair again, so single-agent carboplatin may be an option. Some patients prefer oral to injected drugs, so altretamine, which is well-tolerated in many patients, or etoposide could be considered. Then there are liposomal doxorubicin, gemcitabine, topotecan and vinorelbine. There is even tamoxifen, because hormonal therapy, which is very well tolerated, has response rates in the region of 10–20% in reasonably fit patients.

Response rates to these drugs can be assessed by magnetic resonance imagining and computerized tomography, but a simpler way is to use CA125 levels. Although a serial fall in CA125 levels is used to indicate a response in day-to-day practice, more precise definitions are required in clinical trials. If one investigator uses a 15% fall in CA125 levels to indicate response to treatment and another uses a 50% fall, the response rate will be very different, even among the same group of patients. A lot of work has been done on this, and the definition based on a 50% fall over four samples or a 75% fall over three samples is increasingly being used in clinical trials around the world (Table 2).[7, 8]

Conclusion

There are a number of steps that should be followed in selecting appropriate relapse chemotherapy. The first thing is to determine whether the patient has early (less than six

Table 2 CA125 – definition of response

Response according to CA125 has occurred if either of the following criteria are fulfilled:

- 50% response definition:
  - If there is a 50% decrease in serum CA125 levels from two initially elevated samples, then a 50% response has occurred. The sample showing a 50% fall must be confirmed by a fourth sample (ie four samples required in total).
- 75% response definition:
  - If there has been a serial decrease in CA125 levels of more than 75% over three samples then a 75% response has occurres (ie three samples required in total).

In both 50% and 75% response definitions, the final sample needs to be analysed at least 28 days after the previous sample.

months) or late (more than six months) disease. For early disease, I either give the regimen with the highest response rate (currently weekly platinum plus etoposide) or enter the patient into a trial.

For late disease, I inform the patient of the available options. We have to balance the toxicity of combinations with the slight superiority of others. If a trial drug is available only for first relapse therapy, then I might offer this drug first. If the patient is well and not in a trial, then oral altretamine may be considered for the first relapse, carboplatin for the second relapse, carboplatin or a taxane for the third relapse, liposomal doxorubicin for the fourth relapse, carboplatin or topotecan for the fifth relapse, and possibly weekly cisplatin and etoposide for the sixth relapse. There is also tamoxifen, which can help. With so many treatments to choose from, it is now not uncommon for patients to spend more time in relapse than between initial treatment and relapse.[2]

References

1. Vergote I, Rustin GJ, Eisenhauer EA *et al*. New guidelines to evaluate the response to treatment in solid tumours (ovarian cancer). *J Natl Cancer Inst* 2000; **92**: 1534–5.

2. Blackledge G, Lawton F, Redman C, Kelly K. Response of patients in phase II studies of chemotherapy in ovarian cancer: implications for patient treatment and the design of phase II trials. *Br J Cancer* 1989; **59**: 650–3.

3. Eisenhauer EA, Vermorken JB, van Glabekke M. Predictors of response to subsequent chemotherapy in platinum pretreated ovarian cancer: a multivariate analysis of 704 patients. *Ann Oncol* 1997; **8**: 963–8.

4. Harries M, Gore M. Part II: Chemotherapy for epithelial ovarian cancer – treatment of recurrent disease. *Lancet Oncol* 2002; **3**: 537–45.

5. Meyer T, Nelstrop AE, Mahmoudi M, Rustin GJ. Weekly cisplatin and oral etoposide as treatment for relapsed epithelial ovarian cancer. *Ann Oncol* 2001; **12**: 1705–9.

6. van der Burg ME, de Wit R, van Putten WL *et al*. Weekly cisplatin and daily oral etoposide is highly effective in platinum pretreated ovarian cancer. *Br J Cancer* 2002; **86**: 19–25.

7. Guppy AE, Rustin GJ. CA125 response: can I replace the traditional response criteria in ovarian cancer *Oncologist* 2002; **7**: 437–43.

8. Rustin GJ. Use of CA125 to assess response to new agents in ovarian cancer trials. *J Clin Oncol* 2003. (in press)

Other methods of symptom control

Adrian Tookman, Royal Free Hospital NHS Trust, Edenhall Marie Curie Centre, London

Cancer patients survive longer and palliative care is diversifying. This presents the specialty with new challenges. Specialist palliative care must not only address increasingly complex clinical problems but also be engaged in the process of developing strategies to respond to the widening cancer agenda. The expectations of patients have increased, and they rightly demand that clinicians acknowledge that their needs are broader than those related to their cancer treatment. The emerging supportive care guidance from the Department of Health will enable these issues to be addressed systematically and constructively by cancer networks. Palliative care is an integral component of supportive care, as is symptom control.

The increasing success of modern cancer therapy has led to an increased prevalence of cancer survivors. The issues related to survivorship are of particular relevance to patients with ovarian cancer: patients with advanced ovarian cancer have often been seduced by intensive therapies that result in dramatic initial responses, but the disease itself and the side-effects of these therapies can result in significant disability and long-term sequelae. Chemotherapy-related peripheral neuropathy, problems related to stoma formation, fatigue, pain, ascites and bowel obstruction are a just a few of the physical problems encountered.

Cancer also has a dramatic impact on the emotional, social and sexual domains of a patient's life. Patients who have disease recurrence can become disillusioned when their complex and often arduous treatment regimens have failed and they have to face the realization that they have a life-threatening disease. Patients therefore have complex needs, and the interaction between physical and psychosocial issues must always be considered. Acknowledging this on assessment will lead to an individualized management approach that takes account of all these aspects.

Sexuality

Sexuality is an area that adopts great importance in patients with gynaecological cancer but is often overlooked by clinicians. The issue is complex, focusing on the meaning of femaleness to each individual, and it must be seen in the context of the patient's personality. Whether sexuality issues in patients with advanced cancer should be assessed routinely or reactively in response to open questioning has long been an area for debate. This is illustrated by a study of three cohorts of patients who filled in detailed questionnaires about all aspects of sexuality. One group was from a cancer practice, another was from a palliative-care practice; a comparator group came from primary care. The study demonstrated clearly that all patients have issues relating to their sexuality that they wish to discuss with their professional carers. Sixty per cent of patients with advanced disease would like to have been asked by their professional carer whether they had sexual problems, suggesting that sexuality issues should be elicited at consultation by direct questioning.[1]

Pain

Palliative care plays an important role in the management of pain. The perception that palliation should be reserved for patients who are imminently dying is common and misjudged. By adopting a palliative approach, the quality of pain control will be enhanced for a far wider population of patients. The following groups of patients should be considered for referral to palliative care:

- patients with cancer pain undergoing treatment (surgery, radiotherapy, chemotherapy)
- patients who have pain following definitive treatment
- patients with advanced cancer
- patients with advanced cancer and who are imminently dying
- patients with chronic pain who have advanced, progressive, non-cancer conditions.

Clearly, it is important to treat pain effectively. The majority of patients will gain good relief from the simple strategies recommended by the World Health Organization, which describes a three-step ladder for prescribing analgesics:

1. non-opioid ± adjuvant
2. weak opioid ± non-opioid ± adjuvant
3. strong opioid ± non-opioid ± adjuvant.

These strategies also have a place in patients with complex pathology, as is seen frequently with high-bulk, invasive pelvic disease. Opioid analgesia has always been a mainstay in patients with advanced disease, and morphine has always been considered to be the gold standard. However, some patients cannot tolerate morphine. In particular, patients with ovarian cancer can have specific problems with morphine if there is renal impairment, when morphine elimination can be particularly unpredictable. In these patients, alternative opioids are necessary. Fentanyl does not rely solely on renal excretion and therefore is a good opioid to choose in patients with renal impairment. Hydromorphone, oxycodone and methadone have less active metabolites than morphine and therefore offer advantages over morphine in this situation.

Neuropathic pain is common in infiltrating pelvic disease. Nerve pain is often thought, incorrectly, to be opioid-resistant. It is argued that opioid responsiveness in neuropathic pain should be regarded as relative.[2] Neuropathic pain often requires high doses of opioids and co-analgesics that target the relevant receptors. Following nerve destruction, there may be deafferentation, 'wind-up' and centrally generated pain. Neuropathic pain states are maintained by complex mechanisms involving altered peripheral activity, central excitatory or inhibitory activity, and sympathetic nervous system activity. Another factor that occurs in nerve destruction is disruption of nerve fibres, which can reduce opioid sensitivity through loss of receptors.[3]

Cholecystokinin (CCK) may have a critical role in modulating response to opioid therapy and high levels of CCK are associated with a decline in opioid effectiveness. Conversely, opioid sensitivity is increased by the use of CCK antagonists.[4]

There is increasing evidence that neuropathic pain states involve prolonged activation of the N-methyl-D-aspartate (NMDA) receptor, leading to increased neuronal activity or wind-up.[5] Activation of the NMDA receptor has also been implicated in the development of tolerance to morphine, and a likely site of action for both hyperalgesia and morphine tolerance is the dorsal horn of the spinal cord.[6]

Co-analgesics improve the management of neuropathic pain significantly. With increasing knowledge of the pathways, neurochemistry and receptors involved in pain, it is likely that the management of complex pain will continue to improve. The role of alternative opioids in neuropathic pain is yet to be determined; however, methadone, with its action on a broad range of opioid receptors, serotonin pathways and possibly NMDA receptors, is a reasonable option for use in complex pain with a neuropathic component. The best prescribing patterns of methadone have yet to be determined; it is not an easy drug to administer, but its use in low doses as a co-opioid with morphine offers advantages over using methadone alone (lower doses mean fewer problems with side-effects and accumulation).

Bowel obstruction

Bowel obstruction is common in patients with ovarian cancer. The inadequacy of prolonged conservative management has long been recognized by Baines and Oliver, who published a series of outcomes based on 38 patients with bowel obstruction who were managed medically without nasogastric tubes or intravenous fluids.[7] Pain, colic, nausea and vomiting can be managed by analgesics (opioids), antispasmodics (hyoscine butylbromide) and anti-emetics, usually given subcutaneously by a 24-hour infusion pump. The use of steroids to reverse obstruction and to ease symptoms of nausea, vomiting, pain and distension has been documented by many authors.[8] Since one-third of patients resolve spontaneously, it has always been difficult to determine the precise benefits of steroids, and many palliative-care specialists reserve steroids for resistant cases.

The management of bowel obstruction has changed recently with the addition of octreotide to the therapeutic armamentarium. Octreotide is an antisecretory drug that acts throughout the gastrointestinal tract and has a rapid effect on distension, colicky pain and high-volume vomiting. Guidelines have been developed for the management of bowel obstruction in several units and many now use octreotide early on in management. Rarely, resistant symptomatic cases may require consideration of stenting or venting gastrostomy.[9] When medical management is appropriate, simple guidelines can be implemented that, hopefully, will improve outcomes.

Ascites

Ascites has always been a difficult symptom to manage and management strategies are inconsistent. Again, guidelines may improve management and certainly will provide a way of judging which strategy should be most beneficial. It appears that it is safe to drain ascites without clamping, which will shorten the time that the drainage tube is left *in situ*. This is obviously an advantage to the patient; it may result in fewer infective complications and may shorten in-patient time.[10] However, the management of ascites remains unsatisfactory; diuretics seem to be successful in only a few patients and patients who require frequent taps rapidly become unwell, fatigued and hypoalbuminaemic.

An alternative, minimally invasive technique to control ascites would be a great advantage. Peritoneovenous shunts become obstructed and therefore are not often employed. There are some successfully managed cases described in the literature where shunts were made by performing a saphenoperitoneal anastomosis exploiting the natural biological valves in the saphenous vein.[11] There have also been case reports of ascites being managed with octreotide. The mechanism of action of octreotide in ascites may be its antisecretory effect and/or its ability to block somatostatin receptors, which are present in many cancers.[12]

Terminal illness

It is critical to manage the dying patient well. Terminal illness and end-of-life care continues to be managed badly by clinicians and the wider needs of the patient and her family are often ignored. It is important, therefore, to manage this phase of the illness proactively. The use of guidelines and/or checklists (see Table 1) ensures that the fundamental needs of the patient and her family are addressed.

All clinicians in all specialties should be equipped with the skills to manage dying patients, since this would reduce unnecessary distress and suffering in patients and their families. Specialists in palliative care have a responsibility to educate these clinicians about the care of the dying patient and to work with them to manage difficult cases. A bad death is not only distressing for the patient and family, but also results in unfulfilled, dissatisfied staff.

Table 1 Checklist for managing patients who are imminently dying

	Yes	No	Varies
1. Is the patient likely to die in the next 48 hours?			
2. If appropriate, has this deterioration been communicated with the patient?			
3. If appropriate, have you discussed the use of life-prolonging measures (eg nutrition, hydration, antibiotics) with the family and/or carers?			
4. Has the CPR status been documented? (Trust guidelines)			
5. Does the patient wish to remain in hospital?			
6. Have the spiritual needs been assessed and addressed?			
7. Is the patient comfortable?			
8. Ongoing management: – is medication available for symptom management? – has unnecessary medication been stopped? – is medication administered by an appropriate route? – is there medication prescribed for crises?			

Modified from *The Care of the Dying Checklist*. North London Palliative and Supportive Care Network, 2003.

Conclusion

Supportive care, the management of patients with non-cancer conditions, rehabilitation in cancer care and the expanding cancer agenda are all part of the diversifying practice in palliative care. Whether the specialty is resourced well enough to address all these issues remains to be seen. Hopefully, by working collaboratively, palliative-care clinicians and gynaecological cancer specialists will enable all patients with palliative care needs to receive improved quality of care.

References

1. Ananth H, Jones L, King M, Tookman A. The impact of cancer on sexual function: a controlled study. *Palliat Med* 2003; in press.

2. Portenoy RK, Foley KM, Inturrisi CE. The nature of opioid responsiveness and its implications for neuropathic pain: new hypotheses derived from studies of opioid infusions. *Pain* 1990; **43**: 273–86.

3. Besse D, Lombard MC, Zajac JM. Pre- and postsynaptic distribution of mu, delta and kappa opioid receptors in the superficial layers of the cervical dorsal horn of the rat spinal cord: a quantitative autoradiographic study. *Brain Res* 1990; **521**: 15–22.

4. Dickenson AH. Neurophysiology of opioid poorly responsive pain. *Cancer Surv* 1994; **21**: 5–16.

5. Dickenson AH. NMDA receptor antagonists: interactions with opioids. *Acta Anaesthesiol Scand* 1997; **41**: 112–15.

6. Mao J, Price DD, Mayer DJ. Mechanisms of hyperalgesia and morphine tolerance: a current view on their interactions *Pain* 1995; **62**: 259–74.

7. Baines M, Oliver DJ. Medical management of bowel obstruction in patients with advanced malignant disease. *Lancet* 1985; **2**: 990–3.

8. Feuer D, Broadly K. Systematic review and meta-analyses of corticosteroids for the resolution of malignant bowel obstruction in advanced gynaecological and gastrointestinal cancers. *Ann Oncol* 1999; **10**: 1035–41.

9. Brooksbank MA, Game PA, Ashby MA. Palliative venting gastrostomy in malignant intestinal obstruction. *Palliat Med* 2002; **16**: 520–6.

10. Stephenson J, Gilbert J. The development of clinical guidelines on paracentesis for ascites related to malignancy. *Palliat Med* 2002; **16**: 213–18.

11. Pang LA, Low JM, Ng BK, A successful peritoneovenous shunting of ascites using the great saphenous vein. *Ann Acad Med Singapore* 1992; **21**: 701–4.

12. Cairns W, Malone R. Octreotide as an agent for the relief of malignant ascites in palliative care patients. *Palliat Med* 1999; **13**: 429–30.

Index